WITH ALL MY STRENGTH

God's Design for Physical Wellness

Compiled by Branda Polk

LifeWay Press
Nashville, Tennessee

ISBN 0-6330-0586-X

This book is a resource in the Personal Life category of the Christian Growth Study Plan.
Course CG-0538

Dewey Decimal Classification: 613.7
Subject Heading: PHYSICAL FITNESS

Branda Polk, Health Ministry Specialist
Betty Hassler, Editor-in-Chief
Jon Rodda, Art Director
Jimmy Abegg, Illustrator
Joyce McGregor, Editor
Beth Shive, Copy Editor

Unless otherwise indicated, Scripture quotations are from the Holy Bible, *New International Version,* copyright © 1973, 1978, 1984 by International Bible Society

Scripture quotations identified The Message are from Eugene H. Peterson, *The Message: New Testament with Psalms and Proverbs.* copyright © 1995. Used by permission of NavPress Publishing Group, Colorado Springs, Colorado.

Scripture quotations identified NLT are from the Holy Bible, *New Living Translation,* copyright © 1996. Used by permission of Tyndale House Publishers, Inc., Wheaton, Illinois 60189. All rights reserved.

Scripture quotations identified NASB are from the NEW AMERICAN STANDARD BIBLE, © Copyright The Lockman Foundation, 1960, 1962, 1963, 1968, 1971, 1972, 1973, 1975, 1977, 1995. Used by permission.

To order additional copies of this resource: WRITE LifeWay Church Resources Customer Service; One LifeWay Plaza; Nashville, TN 37234-0113; FAX order to (615) 251-5933; PHONE (800) 458-2772; EMAIL to *customerservice@lifeway.com;* ORDER ONLINE at *www.lifeway.com;* or VISIT the LifeWay Christian Store serving you.

Printed in the United States of America

Adult Ministry Publishing
LifeWay Church Resources
One LifeWay Plaza
Nashville, TN 37234-0175

Table of Contents

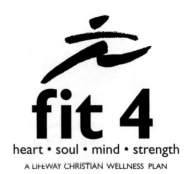

AN INTRODUCTION TO *Fit4*

With All My Strength: God's Design for Physical Wellness is one of four continuing studies in *Fit 4:* **A LifeWay Christian Wellness Plan.** If this is your first *Fit 4* study, welcome to this series which helps individuals achieve wellness one wise choice at a time. Wellness is a lifestyle which includes all four areas of our lives: emotional, spiritual, mental, and physical.

Although this study emphasizes physical wellness, the other areas of wellness are referred to throughout the book because whole-person health involves all that we are. Jesus said it best in Mark 12:30-31—the *Fit 4* theme verses—when He outlined a wellness lifestyle: " 'Love the Lord your God with all your heart and with all your soul and with all your mind and with all your strength. Love your neighbor as yourself.' "

Fit 4 emphasizes three Lifestyle Disciplines to help you live a balanced lifestyle. UPREACH is your relationship to God through daily prayer, Bible reading, and listening to God. OUTREACH is your relationship with others. INREACH is caring for yourself mentally, emotionally, physically, and spiritually. Each week of this study you will find information in the margins which will give you practical suggestions for implementing each of these disciplines daily.

Since our emotions are housed in a body which requires proper food and nutrition to function properly, you will also find in each week a helpful suggestion from our friend Professor Phitt, one of the hosts in the *Fit 4* videos that accompany the two basic courses. These suggestions, found in the margin of each week's reading, will guide

you as you make wise choices in exercise and nutrition. Your *Accountability Journal* will be your friend on your wellness journey. On pages 6-10 you will find information on how to use the *Journal* to track your exercise and food choices for the next 12 weeks. Record your exercise to see patterns, make changes, and set goals to improve your fitness level. Record the food you eat so you become aware of the types and amounts of your daily choices. For more information on making these wise choices, consult pages 14-22 of your *Journal*.

Your group will support your wellness journey. While you encourage and support others, they will do the same for you. Your facilitator will also encourage you as you journey toward mental wellness. Plan to be present for each group session. Contribute your ideas, ask questions, and seek answers from other group members' struggles, victories, and life experiences.

For additional information on a wellness lifestyle, consider being part of a *Fit 4* basic course. *Fit 4 Nutrition* is a 12-week course that will help you apply the *Fit 4* Guidelines for Healthy Eating. *Fit 4 Fitness* is a 12-week course that will help you develop your own personalized fitness plan.

You will also want to participate in the other three continuing studies: *Fit 4 With All My Heart: God's Design for Emotional Wellness,* 0-6330-0583-5; *Fit 4 With All My Soul: God's Design for Spiritual Wellness,* 0-6330-0585-1; and *Fit 4 With All My Mind: God's Design for Mental Wellness,* 0-6330-0584-3. Information about ordering these and other *Fit 4* resources is found on page 8.

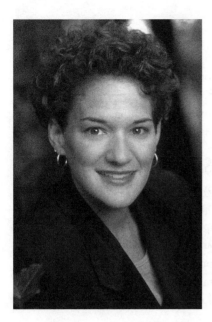

ABOUT THE COMPILER

Branda Polk is the *Fit 4* Coordinator at LifeWay Christian Resources in Nashville, Tennessee. After receiving her Bachelor of Science degree in exercise science with a minor in nutrition, Branda began working in the fitness industry and, to date, has 13 years of experience as a certified personal trainer and fitness instructor. Branda has a passion to help believers understand the value of physical stewardship to life and ministry. Out of this passion she spearheaded the team that created *Fit 4: A LifeWay Christian Wellness Plan*. She is a health writer and speaker on a wide variety of health-related issues and leads wellness conferences nationally and internationally.

Branda is a member of the worship team for her church. In her off time Branda enjoys music, photography, and Little League baseball with her husband, Steve, and their two sons, Jessep and Bryant. They live in Hendersonville, Tennessee.

ABOUT THE STUDY

With All My Strength: God's Design for Physical Wellness is intended as a group study over a 12-week period. The first week's group session will give you an overview of *Fit 4: A LifeWay Christian Wellness Plan*. During this session, you will complete the video viewer guide on page 7.

During the following 10 weeks, you will read each week's content and complete the learning activities which are marked with the *Fit 4* logo ( ). Read the week's material at your own pace. Make sure you complete the reading before the weekly group session. The learning activities provide practice and review for the concepts you will learn. They also improve retention of what you read. A Verse to Know at the beginning of each week will enable you to commit to memory specific verses which will aid you in your wellness journey.

In the margins you will read suggestions for implementing the three Lifestyle Disciplines of *Fit 4*: UPREACH, OUTREACH, INREACH. You will also find helpful advice from our friend Professor Phitt, one of the video hosts from the *Fit 4* basic courses. Professor Phitt will give suggestions for exercise and nutrition choices. The *Accountability Journal* accompanying this book will also encourage you in your wellness journey.

A Leader Guide on pages 103-111 provides the group facilitator with specific information for beginning and conducting a class using *With All My Strength*. Session 11 (week 12) of this study is a group session which provides an opportunity for members to evaluate progress toward goals, set new goals for maintaining a wellness lifestyle, and make plans for participating in other *Fit 4* or discipleship studies.

Remember our *Fit 4* motto: Wellness is achieved one wise choice at a time.

ABOUT THE CONTRIBUTORS

Branda Polk enlisted the following specialists to each write a portion of this study. They have expertise in a variety of disciplines related to health and fitness.

Week 1: Total Wellness

Branda Polk (see page 5)

Week 2: Managing Weight

Julie Opp, MS, RD is a Registered Dietitian with 20 years experience. Julie earned her bachelor's degree in Nutrition and MS in Nutrition and Food Systems Management. She has worked in Food Service Management, as a Nutritionist for the Women, Infant, and Children (WIC) Program, and as a dietetic consultant with long-term care facilities. Julie counsels individuals in weight management. Julie lives in Jamestown, North Dakota.

Week 3: Supplements

Marjorie Jarrett, RD, is an outpatient dietitian at Baptist Center for Health and Wellness in Nashville, Tennessee. She loves spending time with her family, reading, cooking, and serving in the Children's Worship Ministry at her church. Marjorie lives in Hendersonville, Tennessee.

Week 4: Strength Training

John Latham, M.S. is an exercise physiologist and advisory panel member for *Fit 4: A LifeWay Christian Wellness Plan*. He holds certifications by the American College of Sports Medicine, National Strength and Conditioning Association, and the American Association of Lifestyle Counselors and has over 12 years experience in corporate wellness. John lives in Knoxville, Tennessee.

Week 5: Fitness Options

Chad Hendley is a Certified Clinical Exercise Specialist(R) American College of Sports Medicine; and Wellness Coordinator, Satilla Regional Medical Center in Waycross, Georgia. He serves as a member of the *Fit4* expert panel.

Week 6: Eating Disorders

Kelly Preston, RN, MSN, is Congregational Health Program Coordinator for Baptist Health System of Alabama.

After two hospitalizations and several years of therapy for anorexia nervosa, Kelly often shares her testimony about God's healing work that continues to this day. She lives in Birmingham, Alabama.

Week 7: Managing Stress

Susan Lanford currently serves as a chaplain in the Baptist Health system in Little Rock, Arkansas, and as an instructor in the Baptist Health Schools of Nursing and Allied Health. Susan lives in Little Rock, Arkansas. Prior to that, Susan worked at the Mind-Body Institute through Baptist Hospital System in Nashville, Tennessee. She is an accomplished writer on subjects related to all areas of wellness.

Week 8: Successful Aging

Dr. Michael Parker, LTCR, BCD, DSW, LCSW is Assistant Professor in the School of Social Work at the University of Alabama (UA) and Adjunct Assistant Professor of Medicine, Division of Gerontology and Geriatric Medicine at the University of Alabama at Birmingham (UAB). Dr. Parker is one of ten outstanding faculty scholars selected by The John A. Hartford Foundation of New York City and The Gerontological Society of America.

Col. George F. Fuller, MD, MC, United States Army is Associate Chair, Family Medicine Program, Uniformed Services University of the Health Sciences, Bethesda, Maryland. He is a past White House physician.

Weeks 9, 10: Lifestyle Diseases, CAM Therapies

Charles H. Elliott, PA-C, MPAS, is a freelance writer and speaker through Elliott Medical Communications. He is currently the director of occupational and preventive medicine for the employees of a major energy and chemical company. Charles lives in Hilliard, Ohio.

Leader Guide

Judy Howard is a Bible study teacher for all ages. Judy's love of teaching extends into the community were she serves as a job training counselor assisting people in finding employment. Judy, a retired pastor's wife, lives in Gallatin, Tennessee.

FIT 4 RESOURCES

Fit 4 Plan Kit

Includes two copies of the *Facilitator Guide,* four group session videotapes, promotional/facilitator training video, *Nutrition Starter Kit,* and *Fitness Starter Kit.* 0-6330-0580-0

Fit 4 Nutrition Starter Kit

This 12-week course includes a *Nutrition Member Workbook, Accountability Journal Refill Pack* and three-ring binder, *Wise Choices **Fit 4** Cookbook,* and lunch bag imprinted with **Fit 4** logo. 0-6330-0581-9

Fit 4 Nutrition Member Workbook 0-6330-2883-5

Fit 4 Fitness Starter Kit

A 12-week course that includes a *Fitness Member Workbook, Accountability Journal Refill Pack* and three-ring binder, the **Fit 4** *Workout* video, and exercise bag imprinted with **Fit 4** logo. 0-6330-0582-7

Fit 4 Fitness Member Workbook 0-6330-2010-9

Fit 4 Facilitator Guide

Contains group session plans for facilitating both basic courses. Two copies included in *Plan Kit.* 0-6330-0588-6

Fit 4 Accountability Journal Refill Pack

Space to record meals and exercise activities for 13 weeks. Includes helpful nutritional and fitness information. 0-6330-0589-4

Wise Choices Fit 4 Cookbook

Contains easy-to-prepare recipes, menu planning suggestions, a grocery shopping list, food terms, label-reading instructions, and snack suggestions. 0-6330-0587-8

Fit 4 Continuing Studies

- *With All My Heart: God's Design for Emotional Wellness* 0-6330-0583-5
- *With All My Soul: God's Design for Spiritual Wellness* 0-6330-0585-1
- *With All My Mind: God's Design for Mental Wellness* 0-6330-0584-3
- *With All My Strength: God's Design for Physical Wellness* 0-6330-0586-X

Fit4.com Web Site

Up-to-date nutritional and fitness information, calculators for health assessments, fun quizzes, recipes, and more. Features on all four areas of wellness.

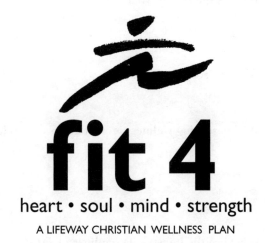

fit 4
heart • soul • mind • strength
A LIFEWAY CHRISTIAN WELLNESS PLAN

TO ORDER COPIES OF THESE RESOURCES:
Write LifeWay Church Resources Customer Service; One LifeWay Plaza; Nashville, TN 37234-0113;
Fax order to (615) 251-5933; Phone 1-800-458-2772; Email to *customerservice@lifeway.com;*
Order online at *www.lifeway.com;* or visit the LifeWay Christian Store serving you.

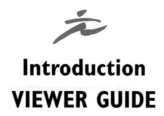

Introduction
VIEWER GUIDE

1. *Fit 4* is designed to help you develop a _____ approach to wellness.

2. What is wellness?

3. The secret to good health is _____.

4. You will use the *Fit 4* guidelines to develop a _____ plan to meet your needs.

5. What is the purpose of your *Fit 4* group?

6. What is the role of your *Fit 4* facilitator?

7. Who is Professor Phitt?

8. Why is seeking wellness important to your relationship with God?

9. What are the Lifestyle Disciplines of *Fit 4?* U_____, O_____, and I_____.

10. Based on what you know thus far, list some personal benefits you can expect to gain from completing this study.

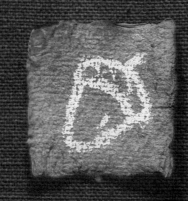

Week One
Total Wellness
Branda Polk

Welcome to this course in the continuing study series of *Fit 4:* **A Christian Wellness Plan.** The theme verses for *Fit 4* are direct words from Jesus found in Mark 12:30-31. Read them in the margin. Jesus told us that the greatest command-ment is loving God, others, and self. Jesus' words help us understand the various aspects of who we are as humans. We're not just emotions or a spirit or a physical body. We're all parts—emotions, soul, mind, and body—wrapped together and intertwined so that no one area acts on its own. We're also relational beings that need other people in our lives. When one area of our person is affected, all the other areas are affected as well. At times, this total person concept is difficult for us to fully understand. But the fact that we cannot fully understand it doesn't make it less true.

With All My Strength specifically addresses the physical aspect of our bodies and shows how they interact with our emotions, mind and soul. Medical science, psychology, and spiritual leaders are beginning to connect and address the total person as Jesus described us. We understand more completely that when we consider physical wellness, we must also address the emotional, mental and spiritual aspects of who we are as well. We are whole people and every event that occurs or change that is made impacts every other area.

 Recall a physical challenge that has occurred in your life. Maybe it was an illness, the birth of a child, a broken bone or other injury, training for a sporting event, or some other physical challenge or event. Write a brief description of this memory below.

_____

_____

Think about the event again. Was it a purely *physical* event? Or did it impact you in other areas of your life? On page 10 write several descrip-tive words telling how you were impacted in the following areas.

VERSES TO KNOW

" ' "Love the Lord your God with all your heart and with all your soul and with all your mind and with all your strength." The second is this: "Love your neighbor as yourself." There is no commandment greater than these.' "
—Mark 12:30-31

Emotions before, during, and after the event: _____

_____

Thoughts before, during, and after the event: _____

_____

Spiritual need or changes before, during, and after the event:_____

_____

Professor Phitt says:
According to the American Heart Association, physical inactivity is as damaging to your heart as smoking. If you are not already exercising, begin by walking 10 minutes at a comfortable pace. Gradually increase your time and speed.

I experienced this interaction of all parts first hand in August 1999. I was diagnosed with level 2, malignant melanoma (skin cancer) from a very small darkened spot on my back. The two millimeter diameter spot was surgically removed the next month, leaving a seven-inch scar on my back. This experience left a very physical scar but it impacted every area of my person. Before the surgery my mind raced from thoughts of denial, to blame, to self-pity. Emotionally I was scared, uncertain, and even angry. My mind was consumed with the small spot on my back and the "what if's" had it not been discovered in time.

During this experience I expressed my love for my family, and I grew in my relationship with my husband as he cared for me. I also grew in my relationship with God. He did a work in my life to break an area of pride. I saw my physical fitness and health as a personal accomplishment. The choices I made to keep myself healthy led to a prideful attitude. I thought I controlled how long I would live. The bout with skin cancer opened my heart so God could remind me that He was the ultimate controller of the days of my life. He held my life in the palm of His hand.

I learned that while caring for my body is important, it's not to be the ultimate focus of my life. The benefits I receive from a healthy body allow me to honor God and not me. God was faithful to heal me and walk with me through it all. My scar is an ever-present reminder of the lessons I learned. Nothing happens to our body that doesn't affect us emotionally, mentally and spiritually. When we grasp how God uniquely created us as whole persons, we can better develop a total wellness plan to accomplish our goals and serve our Lord. Look at the Stress Model (p. 11) to understand how thoughts and emotions impact the total person.

THE CHRISTIAN AND THE PHYSICAL BODY

It's futile to strive for a level of physical fitness or external "perfection" with the belief that fulfillment is found solely in this area of life. Physical beauty is a worldly achievement that leaves us empty. During my years as a fitness instructor and personal trainer, I saw many people attempt to find fulfillment in bigger biceps or flatter abdominal muscles. These trophies left them wanting something that could not be found in the gym. While the external was appealing or could accomplish feats of strength or athletic achievement, the total person was lacking a connection with something greater.

THE STRESS MODEL

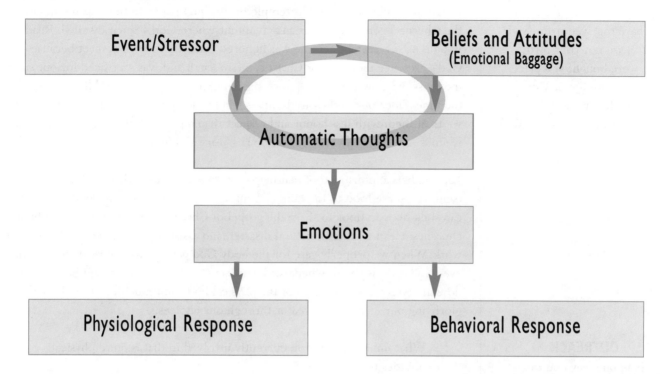

This diagram, adapted from one used at the Mind/Body Medical Institute at Harvard*, shows us how stress works its way into our lives. As **events** come into our awareness, they may or may not become **stressors**. Whether they become stressors depends on the interaction between the event and our personal history, something we can think of as our **beliefs and attitudes** or simply as "emotional baggage." Everyone has baggage! Each individual's baggage is the sum total of the beliefs and attitudes developed in response to past events in his or her life. Some baggage is useful—if you put your hand on a hot stove, it will burn you. Some no longer serve a purpose—if I cross the street without holding someone's hand, I may be hit by a car. Often we continue to hold onto emotional baggage even after it no longer serves us.

Events that take place interact with our beliefs and attitudes and lead to **automatic thoughts**—the unconscious thoughts we have all day long. The majority of our thoughts tend to be negative simply because they try to help us prepare for whatever might happen to us. They also open us to potentially distorted thoughts. Thoughts lead to **emotions**. Emotions are biochemical and physiological as well as mental. These biochemical changes can lead to **physiological** changes that we call stress. They also produce **behavioral** responses.

Notice that **thoughts precede emotions** and that emotions are biochemical changes in your body. This process sets up a cycle or loop in which your mind identifies the biochemical events and labels them as an emotion. Certain biochemical changes may be identified as anger, sadness, happiness, or joy—but the point is that thought precedes emotions. Think happy thoughts, experience happy emotions. Think angry thoughts, feel anger.

Because we each have the ability to change our thoughts, we can change how we feel. We are not helpless victims of our emotions. We have power that we can choose to exercise. Abraham Lincoln has been quoted as saying, "Most people are about as happy as they make up their minds to be." He was right.

* Adapted from Herbert Benson, M.D., and Eileen Stuart, R.N.C., M.S., *The Wellness Book: The Comprehensive Guide to Maintaining Health and Treating Stress-Related Illness* (New York: Simon & Schuster, 1993).

"Do you not know that your body is a temple of the Holy Spirit, who is in you, whom you have received from God? You are not your own; you were bought at a price. Therefore honor God with your body."
—1 Corinthians 6:19-20

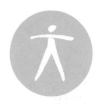

OUTREACH

Find one way you can physically minister to someone else. Write your experience below.

Read 1 Corinthians 6:19-20 in the margin. The apostle Paul clearly states that our bodies are the temple of the Holy Spirit. When we have a relationship with Christ our bodies become His temple or dwelling place. In the Old Testament the tabernacle or temple was an actual tent where God's Spirit dwelled. Read Exodus 40:34-38. The temple was honored and treated with respect because of God's presence there. Since Christ came to earth and was sacrificed for our sin on the cross, we now have the opportunity to have the Spirit of God living in us all the time. Since our bodies are temples where the Spirit of God lives, why should we treat them with less honor and respect than a physical building? As believers we must use the body He gave us for His glory and honor.

Your body is a ministry tool that helps you to accomplish what God intends. Your hands can serve food to the hungry. Your arms can hold a crying child. Your legs can walk door to door to share the gospel of Christ. A strong, fit body can build churches, clean-up after a natural disaster, and assist the sick or elderly with yard work. When we properly care for the body God gave us we are ready to do whatever God calls us to do, whenever He calls us to do it. This concept has little to do with external glorification of the physical body and much more to do with glorifying our marvelous Creator through our choices.

What ministries are you currently involved in that require physical abilities to accomplish?
- ❏ Working with preschoolers or children in Sunday School
- ❏ Taking the youth group to camp, retreats, or other outings
- ❏ Weekday ministries to the homebound or other groups
- ❏ Other (list) _____
- ❏ None

Check the physical abilities necessary to complete this ministry.
- ❏ Strong arms
- ❏ Strong legs
- ❏ Flexible joints
- ❏ Sitting and standing repeatedly
- ❏ Lifting heavy objects
- ❏ Cardio-respiratory (heart/lungs) endurance
- ❏ Strong back
- ❏ Sustained energy
- ❏ Climbing ladders
- ❏ Climbing stairs
- ❏ Balance

God uniquely created your body for a purpose. All of us have a variety of strengths that are valuable in the kingdom of God. Psalm 139 is a powerful passage describing the intimate detail of your creation by God. He didn't make any mistakes in your physical design. As believers our responsibility is to be good stewards of everything God has given us, including our physical bodies, and to seek to honor Him in every area of your life.

PURPOSE OF *WITH ALL MY STRENGTH*

The purpose of this study is multi-dimensional. First, this study highlights various areas of physical health to provide up-to-date information about each topic. Second, this study provides helpful resources for each topic should you desire further information. Third, this study gives helpful information so believers can develop an informed opinion on these topics from a biblical point of reference. Finally, this study equips believers with additional tools for developing a healthful lifestyle that honors God. The basics of developing a healthy eating plan and balanced fitness plan are found in the ***Fit 4*** *Nutrition* and *Fitness* courses.

The *Accountability Journal* provided with this study is a valuable tool on your wellness journey. If you are familiar with this record-keeping system from the *Fitness* and *Nutrition* studies, continue to use it to chart your wellness goals. If not, consider using the *Accountability Journal* on a daily basis to help you reach your goals. Instructions for using the *Accountability Journal* are found on pages 7-9. Recording the amount and types of food that you eat helps you become aware of your food intake. Keeping the weekly journal page up-to-date will enable you to identify areas for improvement and ways to eat the right amount to accomplish your goals. Research has shown that recording food choices can lead you to reduce the amount you eat by 500–1500 calories per day. In turn, recording your activity habits is a powerful motivational tool to get you out of your chair and into action.

> **NOTE:** *With All My Strength* **is not intended to be a diagnostic tool for any of the subjects addressed in the following chapters. Always consult your medical professional for personalized information that is specific to your health situation. Do not make changes in your health plan simply based on this information. Consider this study as a launch pad for discussing relevant issues with your healthcare provider.**

USING THIS STUDY EACH WEEK

This study is a compilation of subjects that offer a broad scope overview of certain topics that can be helpful to everyday life. During each week you will find biblical references in the margins that will encourage deeper Bible study. The Bible does not specifically address many of the topics in this book so we must rely on the strong biblical principles in God's Word. The Bible is rich with truths on which we can build our whole lives and make wise decisions. Combine biblical truth with the revealed truth found in these areas of health to avoid the ebb and flow of cultural fads that lead us down a dangerous path. Use wisdom and discernment when it comes to making health decisions. Read the suggested Scriptures found in the margins and answer the questions related to that Scripture.

This study is not intended to be your only source of spiritual devotion each day. If you are already involved in another daily devotional tool, continue to use it. If you are not reading another devotional aid, turn to page 95 and begin with today's date reading the Bible through. It's always a good time to start.

These professionals who wrote each week's material were prayerfully selected and are strong Christians with an interest in helping believers be totally well. You will read personal testimonies, scientific information, checklists, and practical suggestions related to each topic. Did you stop to read the list of contributors on page 6? Look for answers to the following questions:

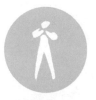

INREACH
When is the last time you had a complete physical check-up from your doctor? If it has been more than one year, schedule an appointment this week.

Week 1—**Total Wellness:** What is a total wellness concept that applies to our physical health?
Week 2—**Managing Weight:** What is the best weight management plan?
Week 3—**Nutritional Supplements:** Are herbs and vitamin/mineral supplements necessary for good health?
Week 4—**Strength Training:** How do I develop a strength training plan to reach my wellness goals?
Week 5—**Fitness Options:** What options are available and most effective?
Week 6—**Eating Disorders:** What are the characteristics of eating disorders?
Week 7—**Managing Stress:** What are the two types of stress?
Week 8—**Successful Aging:** What is the truth about aging? Can I improve my chances of living a longer, healthier life?
Week 9—**Lifestyle Diseases:** What role do my choices play in determining if I get heart disease or cancer? Is obesity a genetic disease?
Week 10—**Complementary and Alternative Medicines and Therapies:** Is a complementary therapy the right method for my health challenges?

ASSESS YOUR CURRENT WELLNESS

In the Appendix on pages 89-94 you will find a "Total Wellness Assessment" that will help you know your stronger and weaker areas so that you will know where you are on your wellness journey. This is not a medical diagnostic tool, but it offers a good guide to know where you are doing well and suggests some areas that may need improvement. To get an accurate picture, honesty with yourself is vital. Some of the statements will be easy to evaluate. Others will take thoughtful and prayerful consideration. Allow God to show you truth about yourself through this assessment. You will not be asked to share this information with anyone. **Complete this assessment before the next group session.**

ESTABLISH YOUR GOALS

Where do you want to go? What do you want to accomplish? In answering these questions you begin the process of establishing goals. Goals are the road markers on the wellness journey that help focus, motivate, and plan our progress. Achieving goals gives opportunity to celebrate accomplishment and set new goals. Slow progress toward a goal or lack of motivation to achieving a goal gives opportunity to re-evaluate the goal. Is this a goal God desires for you to achieve? Do you have the necessary knowledge, support, and plan to achieve this goal? Do you want to achieve this goal? Evaluating goals and aligning them with what God desires for you will help motivate you to continue, despite unexpected circumstances.

When setting your goals, begin with a big picture perspective to give you a long range point of view. Ask yourself: *Do I want to be healthy and active for the rest of my life? What activities do I want to continue doing for the rest of my life? Where to I want to be in 10 years?* These markers become your mileposts for establishing your long-term and short-term goals. Long-term goals are those things you would like to accomplish in the next three to five years. Now break your long-range goals into short-range goals which you can accomplish in the next six months to three years. Then shorter term goals—small markers to accomplishing these goals— can be set to complete in weeks or months. The pattern you use to establish your goals is up to you. The more detailed you are, the more progress you will see on your wellness journey.

Properly defining your goals will create a solid framework. Consider setting **"S.M.A.R.T."** goals. Your goals are:
- Specific: Establish goals that clearly state what you desire to accomplish. An example of a specific goal is "I will lower my cholesterol." A non-specific goal would be "I will get healthy."
- Measurable: Quantify the amount to measure your progress. An example of a measurable goal: "I will lower my cholesterol by 20 points."
- Attainable: Is this a goal you can attain? If your cholesterol is already in a healthy range, is it necessary or possible for you to decrease it by 20 points? Or is it possible to lower your cholesterol 20 points in 2 months?
- Realistic: "Is this goal a wish or one I am willing to work toward?" Having goals that are real to you will motivate you to accomplish them.
- Tangible and Time-Oriented: Tangible goals are not coerced by someone else. Wrapping your goal with a time line completes your chart toward progress.

An example of a lifetime goal: "I will remain active and strong as I age so I can continue to serve God in a wide variety of ways."

An example of a SMART long-term goal would be: "I will complete my college degree in the next five years."

An example of a SMART short-term goal would be: "I will lower my cholesterol from 210 to 190 in 12 months."

During this week, use your quiet time to pray about the goals you would like to set. Allow God to direct your thoughts so the goals you establish are for His glory. Ask God to show you the steps He desires you to take to accomplish these goals. Philippians 4:13 says, "I can do everything through Him who gives me strength." When you allow God to be in the middle of your goal setting, then you can confidently walk in His strength to accomplish these goals.

Remember to consult your health provider before making drastic changes in your lifestyle. Then, seek to personally apply the information you learn. Allow this information to move you closer to accomplishing your goals and improving your ministry opportunities. As you continue to make changes in your lifestyle, avoid focusing on doing everything perfectly. Striving for perfection in our choices and habits is an unrealistic trap that leads to guilt, shame, and feelings of failure. Only Jesus was perfect in this world. Look for ways to make progress on your wellness journey. Progress toward your goals, no matter how small, is success. Progress, not perfection, is the key to success on our wellness journey.

Each chapter may not apply directly to you, but learning the information may benefit you later in life or be used to reach out to someone else. God may open doors where you can minister to others through the knowledge you have gained. Avoid

UPREACH
Read Psalm 16:1-11.
1. Who provides counsel for you?

2. What are 3 benefits of putting the Lord first in your life (see vv. 8-9)?

3. Who will make your path known to you?

pushing others toward making changes. Live a life that will honor God and set a positive example. Be ready to share the message of hope provided through a relationship with Christ. Your *Fit 4* group session will offer other opportunities to share and learn from each other. Commit to pray for each person in your class during the week. Encourage others with affirmations of progress. Remind each other that progress, not perfection, is the key to success on our wellness journey.

A CHALLENGE FOR THIS STUDY

As you read each chapter challenge yourself to complete the *Lifestyle Disciplines* of *Fit 4*—UPREACH, OUTREACH, and INREACH. These *Lifestyle Disciplines* give a framework for developing a wellness lifestyle that honors God. Look again at the Verses to Know for this week (Mark 12:30-31). Can you identify the Lifestyle Disciplines in this passage? Write them below.

UPREACH: _____

OUTREACH: _____

INREACH: _____

In each chapter you will have the opportunity to grow in your walk with God. As you read your Bible each day and spend time with God you will encourage spiritual growth. As you learn the biblical truth involved in each topic you will grow in your understanding of the amazing body that God created for you. Seek to honor God with your choices and grow in your personal relationship with Him.

Do you personally know Jesus Christ as your Savior? Do you know for sure that you will spend eternity with Him in heaven when your days on earth have ended? Jesus was the perfect sacrifice for our sin. If you are not sure about your relationship with Christ, you can know Him personally. Turn to page 102 and read how to become a Christian. God loves you and desires to have a relationship with you. This is the most important decision you will make on your wellness journey. Wellness apart from Christ is impossible. If you do know Christ as Savior, turn to page 102 and review the steps to becoming a Christian. Be ready to share your faith in Christ with others.

May God richly bless you as you continue on your wellness journey with Him— one wise choice at a time.

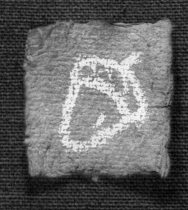

Week Four
Strength Training
John Latham

Once thought to be only for athletes or those wanting to compete in bodybuilding, the last 15 years has seen strength training rise to become one of the most popular fitness activities for people of all ages. The benefits of strength training—also called weight training, weight lifting, resistance training, and pumping iron—seems to be only surpassed by the number of ways you can work your muscles! As the research continues to pour in, major scientific organizations are realizing the need to promote strength training for muscular fitness just as adamantly as cardio-respiratory training for the heart and lungs. Position stands and guidelines distributed by the American College of Sports Medicine now recommend strength training at a minimum of two days per week as part of a comprehensive fitness plan.

Development of muscular strength and endurance is both skill related and health related. For athletes and "weekend warriors," developing strength and speed through strength training can greatly enhance performance. It's hard to drive a golf ball, play full court basketball, hit a softball, or kick a soccer ball without muscular strength and endurance. A stronger athlete is almost always the better athlete.

For the average population, maintaining at least a normal level of strength is extremely important to maintaining function and quality of life as one ages. Adults who don't engage in some type of strength training lose on average ½ pound of muscle every year past age 30. Muscle weakness or imbalance can result in poor posture, abnormal gait, and low back pain, one of the most common health ailments in the United States. If you have already completed the *Fit4* Fitness study, then you have been introduced to some basic values of strength training for muscular strength and endurance.

- Prevents and rehabilitates injury
- Assists in weight control
- Helps prevent and treat osteopenia/osteoporosis
- Maintains quality of life and functionality during aging
- Improves athletic performance

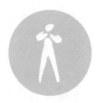

INREACH
Complete the "Physical Activity Readiness" Questionnaire on page 12 of the *Accountability Journal*. If you answer yes to more than two statements, consult your physician for a physical exam.

Read Colossians 1:9-14.

1. What four characteristics are shown in a person who lives a life worthy and pleasing to the Lord (vv. 10-12)?

1. _____

2. _____

3. _____

4. _____

2. What have we been rescued from and brought into by Christ?

3. Thank God for this gift of forgiveness and redemption.

This chapter will take you farther on your strength journey by looking more in depth into the principles and program design of this important component of total wellness. Possibly you have little or no strength-training experience and yet are a healthy adult. Discussing strength training for special populations is beyond the scope of this chapter. If you have special needs, you can certainly tailor the principles I'll share to your specific condition. Always seek the advice of your medical care professional before beginning any strength training program.

Let's get started by nailing down some basic strength-training lingo. Next, we'll explore basic strength-training principles, and then finish up with design and examples of various strength-training routines.

BASIC DEFINITIONS

Here are some basic terms used in describing strength-training programs and principles.

Resistance: What is being used for the muscles to lift or work against in order to elicit a training effect. Resistance can come from a variety of forms such as free weights, machines, rubber bands, body weight, medicine balls, milk jugs filled with water, or even manual resistance from a workout partner.

Repetitions: One complete movement of a strength-training exercise. It normally consists of lifting and lowering the resistance; often referred to as "reps."

Set: A group of repetitions performed in succession without stopping. A set can be made up of any number of repetitions depending on the needs and goals of the participant, however, a typical set usually ranges from 1 to 15 repetitions.

Rest period: Recovery between multiple sets of the same exercise and between different exercises. The length of the rest periods is primarily determined by program goals.

Active Rest: A brief time of 1-2 weeks where the strength trainer takes a break from his/her routine but continues eclectic physical activity for a physiological and psychological break. For example, someone may just go into the weight room and do what they feel like doing. Or the participant may elect to stay completely out of the weight room and play a vigorous sport instead. Progress of the past training cycle is reviewed and training routine is often changed to continue progress toward short term goals.

Repetition Maximum: Abbreviated as RM; the maximal number of repetitions per set that can be performed at the selected resistance with proper lifting technique. Therefore, a set at a certain "RM" implies the set is performed to volitional fatigue. For example, if a person can lift 50 pounds only one time without breaking proper form or technique then 50 pounds would be his/her 1 RM. The same person might be able to lift a lighter weight of 35 pounds for 8 repetitions, but not 9. So, 35 pounds would be his/her 8 RM.

Concentric Phase: When a weight is being lifted, the involved muscles are usually shortening. The part of an exercise in which the muscles are shortening is called the concentric phase of the exercise.

Eccentric Phase: When lowering a weight in a controlled manner, the involved muscles are usually lengthening, but are still under tension. If the muscles did not continue to contract during the lowering or eccentric phase, the weight would fall abruptly back to the starting position. This eccentric phase is also sometimes referred to as the negative part of the exercise. Eccentric contractions are the primary cause of muscle soreness but are also primarily responsible for producing strength gains.

PRINCIPLES OF PROGRAM DESIGN

Keep the terminology you just learned in your mind and refer back to it as we learn the basic principles of strength training and program design. Later, you'll see examples of how to manipulate these variables to achieve your personal programs goals as well as to keep variety in your strength-training routine.

Overload

A good understanding of the overload principle must be at the heart of any strength-training program. The overload principle simply states, if you want to improve the musculoskeletal system, then you must place an unaccustomed load on it. Without overload, your strength-training program will not produce results. For beginners, overload is almost automatic. Someone who has been doing relatively nothing can easily add activity to provide an overload! Any amount of overload will produce results, but heavier resistance loads at or near maximal effort will produce significantly greater training effects. One must take caution to gradually increase training overload (intensity) over time in order to prevent injury and burnout. This brings us to our next training principle.

Progression

Let's say you begin a strength-training program, and one of your exercises is a biceps curl. Curling 20 lbs. is too easy so you start with 50 lbs. which is more challenging and certainly provides an overload stimulus. You are very faithful and perform your routine three times per week. Over time, your biceps adapt to the 50 lb. load, and before you know it, what used to be challenging is now relatively easy and is no longer providing an overload. You have become accustomed to the 50 lb. load. When the muscles adapt to a given load there is no further increase in muscular strength and endurance. In order to continue progressing, you'll need to manipulate certain variables to continue providing overload. This is where the principle of progression comes in. Progression is systematically increasing the demands placed on the muscles in order to continue improving.

These two principles of progression and overload are often coupled together in the literature as "progressive overload." The often used Greek legend of Milo of Crotona illustrates how these two principles work together. According to legend, Milo began hoisting a baby ox onto his shoulders and climbing a hill. As the baby

OUTREACH

Use your strength every day. Look for ways to perform random acts of kindness. Volunteer your services and expect nothing in return. Ideas include: Help a mother with small children or elderly person carry and load groceries; mow a neighbors lawn without them knowing you did it; help a fellow traveler with luggage; assist a co-worker with a load of paper work or a computer case.

ox grew, Milo continued his ritual. Each day, little by little, Milo adapted to the weight of the growing ox until it was full grown. He then demonstrated his great strength at an Olympiad by hoisting the full grown ox onto his shoulders and carrying it around the stadium!

I suggest something besides oxen for your resistance! But this story should help you understand that in order to improve, you must progressively challenge the muscular system beyond its regularly accustomed level. A little today and a little more tomorrow! The importance of the overload and progression principles can't be overemphasized if you want to make gains in your strength-training program.

There are several ways progressive overload can be introduced into your program:
1. You can increase the resistance. With free weights or machines, simply add more weight. With rubber bands, different colors are available which offer increased resistance.
2. You can increase the number of repetitions.
3. You can increase the number of sets.
4. You can shorten your rest periods.

Later, we'll look at some sample programs that show how to manipulate these variables to build progressive overload into your strength-training program. But first, let's continue looking at a couple of additional principles you'll want to consider to tailor your program to your specific needs and goals.

Specificity

The principle of specificity states that all training adaptations are specific to the stimulus applied, to the area of the body being trained, and in the manner in which you train. For example, training the legs will have little or no effect on the arms, shoulders, and torso muscles and vice versa. Muscular strength is best developed using heavier weight with fewer repetitions, and muscular endurance is best developed using lighter weight with higher repetitions. While both are developed under each condition to some extent, the principle of specificity states that each loading scheme favors a more specific type of neuromuscular development. The following chart represents specificity in the development of muscular strength and endurance on a continuum. As repetition maximum (RM) increases, the emphasis shifts from strength to endurance. Low RM indicates strength training; high RM indicates endurance training.

INREACH

Are you aware of your specific goals? Review the goals you set in week 1. Modify your goals if necessary based on what you have learned so far in this study. Develop a strength training plan that will help you reach your goals.

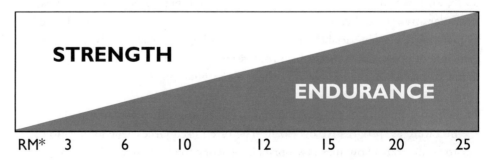

STRENGTH

ENDURANCE

| RM* | 3 | 6 | 10 | 12 | 15 | 20 | 25 |

* Repetition Maximum (refer back to definitions)

While the principle of specificity is probably more important for athletes than for the average person, it certainly needs to be considered when tailoring your program toward specific needs and goals. If someone has low-back pain, then skewing his strength-training program with exercises to promote mid-truck stability would be specific to his needs. Likewise, someone who unloads heavy packages may want to skew her program toward developing both muscular strength and endurance, particularly for the upper body. A person with osteoporosis or osteopenia would benefit by choosing and emphasizing exercises to strengthen the bones and joints.

Variation

Like specificity, the principle of variation is not as important for the beginner as for the seasoned strength trainer and athlete. Nevertheless, altering one or more program variables over time not only allows the training program to remain optimal but also helps alleviate monotony and boredom. In recent years, a concept of variation that has taken strength training by storm is periodization. A typical periodized workout plan would call for an initial high training volume of low intensity favoring muscular endurance (lighter weight, lots of sets and/or lots of reps, shorter rest periods)—more of a circuit type training approach. As training progresses, volume decreases and intensity increases to maximize muscular strength and power (heavier weight, less sets, less reps, longer rest periods)—more of a classical training approach. This cycling of training is repeated several times each year with a couple of weeks of active rest interspersed between training cycles.

Vary your program from workout to workout. For example, a typical Monday, Wednesday, Friday routine may rotate between heavy, moderate, and lighter resistance loads. A systematic changing of exercises which work the same muscle group in a different manner (swapping squats for a lunge, changing from a barbell curl to a dumbbell curl, changing from free weight to machines) also applies the principle of variation. Once you learn the basics, the possible variations are endless!

Sequence

Workouts should begin with the largest muscle groups and proceed to the smallest. Training the large muscle groups first causes the greatest overall stimulation for muscle growth. Once you progress your training to volitional fatigue, you will find it impossible to exhaust larger muscle groups if smaller muscles serving as a link between the resistance and large muscles have already been fatigued. An example would be working the triceps to exhaustion before working the chest on the bench press. The triceps are a smaller muscle group than the chest but act as a link between the chest and the resistance. Fatiguing the triceps first would not allow the full stimulation of the chest muscles. For best results the exercise sequence should be as follows: hips, legs, chest, upper back, arms, waist, and lower back.

Remember that these basic principles of strength training aren't set in stone. As you progress in your training, you may want to bring a lagging body part to the forefront of your workout in order to work it while you are fresh. Changing the order of your exercise routine occasionally is also a way of implementing the variation principle you learned about in the last section.

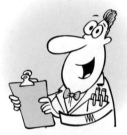

Professor Phitt says:
Fuel your strength training plan with quality calories. Eat lean, low-fat protein, complex carbohydrates and healthy fats to provide energy for your workout and rebuilding your muscles.

INREACH

Muscle is 75 percent water.
Drinking 64 ounces of water
each day will keep you
hydrated and strong.

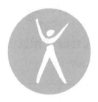

UPREACH

Read Judges 13:5 and
16:4-22. Why did Samson
lose his strength?

How is your strength
affected when you obey God?
When you disobey God?

Frequency

Unlike cardio-vascular training which can be done every day, frequency of strength training will primarily depend on the design of your program. Rest at least 48 hours but not more than 96 hours between strength-training sessions. The American College of Sports Medicine recommends that all healthy adults strength train a minimum of two times per week. Since most of us are sedentary, this training would do wonders in preventing and/or slowing the progression of lifestyle ailments associated with inactivity and aging. As time permits, add strength training to a third time per week. A typical 3-day novice routine is Monday, Wednesday, Friday full-body workouts with about 48 hours of rest between strength sessions.

More advance trainers perform split routines working the upper body on Mondays/Thursdays, and lower body on Tuesdays/Fridays while taking Wednesdays off. This allows for about 72 hours rest for the targeted muscles. Contrary to popular thinking, an advanced strength trainer does not need more exercise but rather less exercise at a higher level of intensity. His or her philosophy should become "work hard, work brief, then rest and grow!" Balance this with your needs and abilities.

PUTTING IT ALL TOGETHER

Whew! Now that we've examined the terminology and basic principles, we are ready for more practical application. Let's look at some sample programs that build in the principles of overload, progression, specificity, variation, sequence, and appropriate frequency.

Let's meet Mike, a typical 43 year-old business executive who travels a lot and has no leisure time physical activity. A recent doctor's visit showed he is apparently healthy but moderately overweight. Mike has noticed that he fatigues easily, and activities of daily living like mowing the lawn or washing the car basically wipe him out for the rest of the day. More recently, Mike went on a short-term mission trip to help build a church and was so sore after the first day he decided it was time to change some habits. Now, Mike commits to 30 minutes on Monday, Wednesday, and Friday for his workout. He bought some light resistance tubing that he can easily throw in his suitcase when traveling. On page 37 you will find an example of what Mike's program might look like for the first six weeks.

The principles of strength training are designed into Mike's routine. Overload and progression is initially provided by increasing the volume. Weeks 1-3 manipulate the sets and reps and increase total volume from 15 reps, to 20 reps, to 30 reps. Week 4 continues progressive overload by cutting the rest periods in half. Week 5 cuts the rest periods again and increases total volume of the routine to 45 repetitions per exercise.

The routine is specific to Mike's needs because it emphasizes lower intensity and higher repetitions. Not only is this ideal for a beginner, but it will also promote more local muscle endurance. The routine emphasizes the upper back which typically needs attention in those who spend a lot of time at a desk or in a forward shoulder posture.

The sequence is proper because large muscle groups are targeted first. Variation is brought in by manipulating both the volume and rest periods. Mike's frequency of 3 days per week with 48 hours rest between exercise sessions is appropriate. In Week 7 Mike could start his 6-week routine over but progress to a higher load by going to a heavier resistance tubing. His possibilities are endless since he now understands the principles behind proper strength-training design!

MIKE'S STRENGTH TRAINING REGIMEN
WEEK 1
15 reps performed Mon., Wed., Fri.; 60 seconds rest between exercises

Activity	# of Reps
1. Squats	15 reps
2. Lunges	15 steps each leg
3. Calf raises	15 each leg
4. Chest press (w/tubing)	15 reps
5. Seated row (w/tubing)	15 reps each arm
6. Shoulder shrug (w/tubing)	15 reps
7. Lateral raises (w/tubing)	15 reps
8. Chair dips	15 reps
9. Bicep curl (w/tubing)	15 reps
10. Abdominal crunches	15 reps
11. Back extensions	15 reps

See exercise descriptions in Appendix (pp. 99-100).

WEEK 2
Same routine as week 1 with the following changes: perform 2 sets of 10 repetitions of each exercise, 60 seconds rest between sets and exercises

WEEK 3
Same routine as with the following changes: perform 2 sets of 15 repetitions of each exercise, 60 seconds rest between sets and exercises

WEEK 4
Stay with sets and reps of week 3.
Cut rest to 30 seconds between sets and exercises

WEEK 5
Go through routine in a circuit fashion (doing 1 set of 15 reps on each exercise) with as little rest as possible.
Rest 3 minutes and repeat routine in circuit fashion.
Rest 3 minutes, and repeat.

WEEK 6
Active Rest

Now let's consider Sally, a 38-year-old stay-at-home mom. She needs help in losing those last 10-15 pounds from her last pregnancy, and her gym offers childcare. Since Sally is new to weight training, she decides to stay with machines. The gym trainer sets up this routine:

UPREACH
Read the Verse to Know for this week and commit it to memory. Thank God for His healing power.

SALLY'S STRENGTH TRAINING REGIMEN

Consult a health club trainer for orientation to these machines and exercises.

Activity	# of Reps
1. Leg Extension for quadriceps	15 reps
2. Leg Curl for hamstrings	15 steps each leg
3. Adductor/Abductor for inner thighs/outer hips	15 each leg
4. Toe Press for calves	15 reps
5. Upright row for mid-upper back	15 reps each arm
6. Chest press machine for chest	15 reps
7. Lateral raise machine for shoulders	15 reps
8. Cable pressdowns for triceps	15 reps
9. Cable curls for biceps	15 reps
10. Crunch machine for abdominals	15 reps
11. Low back extension machine for lower back	15 reps

WEEK 1
Sally performs 15 repetitions of each exercise learning proper form and technique.

WEEK 2
Now familiar with her routine, she increases the resistance over week 2 so she can do 15 repetitions on each exercise in good form (her 15 RM for each exercise).

WEEK 3
Sally increases the resistance in week 3 so that she can grind out 12 reps in good form but not 13. (This is her 12 RM.)

WEEK 4
Sally continues to progressively increase the resistance on each exercise to her 10 RM. She also adds a second set of each exercise with one minute rest between sets.

WEEK 5
She increases the resistance to her 8 RM for each exercise and performs 2 sets with one minute rest periods. They're really hard, but she knows rest comes next week.

WEEK 6
Active rest.

Sally's routine systematically increases the resistance load and becomes increasingly more intense from week to week; it tends to emphasize more upper body exercises since females typically lack strength there. Like Mike's, Sally's routine moves from large to small muscle groups. However, there is very little to no variation in Sally's routine over the six weeks. After the active rest, she might choose to try a few free weight exercises. Her frequency of 3 days per week is working well.

By understanding the principles of strength training and program design, you can tailor a program for your needs and goals. To keep your program effective, follow the recommendations for Strength Training found on page 98 in the Appendix.

OUTREACH

Recite the Verse to Know for a friend, family member or coworker. Share what you have learned about strength training this week

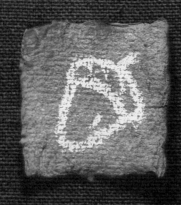

Week Five
Fitness Options
Chad Hendley

Hopefully, you have begun to understand what it means to love God "with all of your strength" (Mark 12:30). God's people must be ready to respond when called into service. Achieving and maintaining physical fitness makes it easier to say *yes*.

The F.I.T.T. principle explains the basics of exercise in very simple terms.
- "F" stands for frequency. How often should we exercise?
- "I" is for intensity. How hard should we push ourselves?
- "T" is for time. How long should we perform any certain exercise?
- The second "T" is for type. What exercises should we do?

Once we determine how much exercise is enough to meet our fitness goals, we can begin experimenting with what types of exercise work best for us. This week we will explore many different exercise options. As you will see, any exercise can work within our F.I.T.T. guidelines. Exercise just needs to be frequent enough, long enough, and intense enough to cause our bodies to respond by getting stronger.

A few years ago, the United States Surgeon General sent out a report stating that sedentary people were actually at a much higher risk for developing certain chronic diseases. These chronic diseases include coronary artery disease, type 2 diabetes, stroke, high blood pressure, and many others. (See week 9, "Lifestyle Diseases" on pp. 73-80.) The Surgeon General concluded that people who increase their physical activity by 15-20 minutes on most days of the week could achieve significant health benefits and improve their quality of life. This study was incredibly important but most people missed it!

With the progress of technology, our lives have become increasingly less physical. As a result of computers, cell phones, and other technological innovations, we don't have to move as much as we did in the past. Most people don't lift, push, pull, walk, or sweat while at work anymore. People now sit for the majority of their work days. We have more instances of back strain, eyestrain, and something new called *Carpal Tunnel Syndrome*. People in our society have to look for opportunities to be more physically active, because our jobs no longer demand it of us.

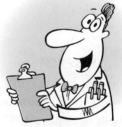

Professor Phitt says:
For additional information about the F.I.T.T. plan, review pages 25-29 of the *Fit 4 Fitness* member workbook and pages 14-17 in your *Accountability Journal*.

Our health has paid the price for our sedentary lifestyles. Obesity is more prevalent than ever before, and so are obesity related diseases such as type 2 diabetes, which is being diagnosed in children as well as adults. On the whole, children, as well as adults, are suffering the consequences of being less physically active

INCREASE YOUR PHYSICAL ACTIVITY/EXERCISE

Physical activity and exercise training aren't necessarily the same things. To increase physical activity, a person only has to find ways to move more often. It's that simple. Take the stairs rather than ride the elevator. Park at the back of a parking lot and walk to the store rather than driving around waiting for that front row person to move. Take a walk around your building on your break rather than hitting the vending machines.

There are many simple ways that we can build activity into our days, and by doing so we can significantly improve our health. To begin our journey through the many exercise options, we should all start by just looking for simple ways to be more active every day. The charts on pages 47-48 illustrate this point very well. Take a close look at the differences in calories used for sedentary activities as compared to the more physical ones.

Walking

Walking remains one of the oldest and greatest forms of exercise. Walking doesn't require any kind of special equipment or place. A person can walk anywhere—a track, a treadmill, or just around his neighborhood. People can even get exercise by walking through a mall or around a department store. Walking is easily adaptable to any environment, indoors or outdoors, and fits well into the basic guidelines for exercise. It's a low-impact exercise, which means that it's easy on your joints. One of the greatest advantages of walking is that it doesn't cost anything!

Pedometers have become a popular tool to help people take more steps each day. A pedometer is a small device that looks much like a beeper. You wear it on your belt, wrist, or on your pocket, and it counts the number of steps you take throughout the day. First, use it to determine how many steps you take each day. Then, try to gradually add more walking into your everyday routine. Pedometers will help motivate you to walk more as you check it several times a day. The cost ranges from 10 to 30 dollars for just a basic model. However, when you add more bells and whistles, the cost may go a little higher.

Running

Running is another tried and true form of exercise. In fact, when someone talks about fitness, the first thing that comes to mind is someone running along a nice scenic road. Runners are the model of physical fitness, mainly because running is difficult. Not everyone is going to be a runner. It takes a lot of discipline and hard work to build up enough stamina to be an endurance runner.

Most exercise specialists would advise people to start walking first before trying to run. Once walking becomes pretty easy, start adding short bouts of running into

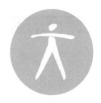

OUTREACH

Invite a person in your class, a coworker, neighbor, or friend to join you for a 30 minute walk.

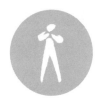

INREACH

Consider investing in a pedometer to determine your number of steps each day. Find them at sports stores or on the Internet for as little as $10. Set a goal to walk at least 5,000 steps a day.

your routine. Gradually begin running more and walking less. Before you know it, you will be that person running along a scenic road, the very picture of fitness.

Running has many of the same advantages of walking. The cost is low, and it can be done almost anywhere. However, running is much more intense. It gets your heart rate much higher than walking. All through the ages, one of the greatest feats of physical prowess has been racing to see who is the fastest or who can run the farthest.

However, running can also take a toll on your body. Running is a high-impact exercise. When you hit the road for a long run, your body takes a great deal of pounding—particularly your ankles, knees, and hips. A gradual approach to running, as described earlier, is the best. Like acquiring a taste for a new food, your body needs to gradually get used to running; once that occurs, you'll be able to go faster and farther, depending on your fitness goals.

Cycling

Cycling is a great exercise, and like walking, is low-impact. For anyone with joint problems, bike riding makes a great exercise option. It takes much of the stress and strain off of your joints. It gets your heart rate up pretty quickly and can really tighten and tone your legs. Cyclists always have very strong legs.

Traditional bikes come in three major categories: cruisers, mountain bikes, and road bikes. Depending upon which type of riding you prefer, chose the right bike. They each have advantages and disadvantages. Stationary bikes are also a great choice, if you prefer indoor exercise. A stationary bike doesn't take up much room and allows you to bike no matter the weather or outside temperature.

Spinning is the most recent cycling craze. Spinning is a term used to describe a cycling class. In a spinning room, you will find several stationary bikes in sort of a semi-circular pattern. An instructor rides along on a bike facing the others and gives instructions to the riders in the class. If you really like to sweat, try a spinning class! It's a great way to jazz up exercising on a stationary bike.

Water Fitness

Water exercise has some great advantages. The water provides a smooth resistance that builds muscle and increases heart rate while giving a total body workout. Perhaps the greatest thing about water exercise is that the buoyancy of water takes away much of the stress on a person's joints. People who can barely move on dry land due to joint pain can get around much easier in a pool. Water fitness is an excellent option for people with orthopedic problems.

Several different types of exercises can be done in the water. The most common is to swim laps. If you've ever watched the summer Olympics, you will recognize this activity. The other form of pool exercise is commonly called water aerobics, typically performed in group classes and in water of four to five feet. An instructor leads the class through various exercises using the water for resistance. Several tools can be

UPREACH
Read 1 John 1:7 the Verse
to Know on page 41.
Commit it to memory.

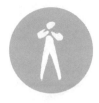

INREACH

Try something new! Select a different form of exercise. Participate three to five times to fully evaluate the exercise. Your body will appreciate and respond to the challenge.

used to enhance the resistance such as webbed gloves and flippers for your feet. Disadvantages to water exercise include the fact that it requires a pool. Most people don't have their own backyard pool; as a result, they may have to pay a membership fee at a fitness facility and attend regular classes.

If you are already a good swimmer, you will not have to work as hard as someone who isn't a seasoned swimmer. If you are trying to build endurance or get your heart rate to a new level, those already swimming may need to find a more challenging activity.

Aerobic Classes

The most popular form of group exercise, aerobic classes are led by an instructor who directs a group of exercisers in different exercise movements. Aerobic classes are typically held in a large open room and use music to set the pace and style. Aerobic classes have evolved over time and include all kinds of variations. The use of several different exercise tools such as hand weights, bands, or steps have made some classes more intense.

The blending of martial arts movements into traditional aerobics classes has created a very popular exercise class called cardio-kickboxing. Various self-defense techniques are used to increase heart rate and keep the interest of participants. These types of group classes also include boxing movements.

Yoga has become very popular. These exercises can be done alone by a single exerciser or in a group. This type of exercise is of Asian descent and involves slow and controlled movements. It increases strength and flexibility by causing the participants to focus and concentrate on their bodies.

Often these classes are linked to spiritual and mental exercises as well as physical. However, some classes only refer to the physical movements. Ask questions before you sign up for a class. Although you can elicit good physical gains, as Christians we must avoid the spiritual implications of Eastern mysticism and meditation. For more information, read the section on yoga included in week 10, "CAM Therapies," on pages 85-86.

Aerobic video tapes are available in most discount stores and multimedia outlets. A number of videos featuring Christian music are available at LifeWay Christian stores and other Christian bookstores. Additional videos can be ordered by mail. Exercising with a tape in your own home is a benefit for those who don't live near a gym or who don't need the support of a group. This approach takes willpower. If you exercise alone, vary the rotation of the tapes and use tapes that also include toning and strength and flexibility exercises.

Competitive Sports

Let's face it. Performing the same exercise day in and day out can get monotonous. Athletic events create competition and cause the competitors to focus on the game rather than the exercise. We run, jump, throw, hit with bats or racquets, or compete against a clock or ourselves. We get caught up in the activity and before we know it, hours have gone by. We are exhausted and don't even realize it.

Sports offer excellent exercise opportunities. Almost every sport can help increase the physical fitness of participants. At the end of this chapter, you will find a chart that shows how many calories are burned during various activities. Many of your favorite sports are there, as well as the activities that we have mentioned thus far. Chose several different options that you enjoy, and go burn some calories.

Exercise Equipment

Fitness centers have many different types of exercise machines. You can also buy them in various sporting goods and department stores. Most are designed for indoor use. Treadmills and stationary bikes, the most traditional pieces of exercise equipment, are the two staples of any fitness center. However, even these main-stays have been improved by technology. Today many bikes and treadmills are connected to television monitors and earphones. You can virtually walk or jog down a scenic path or bike ride in a race—all through the magic of television.

New types of cardiorespiratory exercise equipment include the stair climber or stair stepper. It's basically a staircase on a treadmill. The newcomers on the block in exercise equipment are elliptical trainers or elliptical gliders, which simulate a running motion without the impact of actually jogging. Your feet never leave the platform, or footrest. They move along a circular path. Like a treadmill, skier, and stairclimber combined, elliptical trainers are great exercise machines. While one of its advantages is extremely low impact, those who exercise for bone formation will need impact workouts that the elliptical trainer doesn't provide.

Other new machines routinely appear on the market. These machines can be found in fitness centers or they can be purchased and put in your home. Keep in mind that no magical piece of equipment exists that you only have to use for five minutes a few days a week. Companies make outrageous claims guaranteeing you fast results. Don't be fooled by marketing schemes.

Each of us needs at least 30 minutes of exercise on at least three days a week to maintain good physical fitness, and that is just the minimum. Stick with the proven exercise formulas you have learned in this book and in the ***Fit 4*** *Fitness Member Workbook*. Be sure to include strength training and stretching, vital components of a good workout routine.

Cross Training

Cross training is the practice of changing your exercise routine with different activities. Walk one day and ride a bike the next. Play a sport on occasion, or go for a swim in a pool. Try different activities. Although you will have favorites, you will never know what they are until you experiment. Each activity or exercise has special benefits or improves different areas of the body. For example, some exercises may be more aerobic, whereas others may build more muscle. When you

UPREACH
Read 1 Timothy 4:1-8.
1. What should be the attitude of your heart when you eat good food that God created?

2. Does physical training have value to life on this earth (v. 8)?

3. What type of training has eternal value (v. 8)?

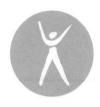

UPREACH
Read Hebrews 12:1-12.

1. Who endured the ultimate "cross" training for our sin? (See v. 2.)

2. What value does discipline have in our lives? Is it easy? Is it worth the effort?

3. What is promised to the lame when they are strengthened (v. 12-13)?

combine these activities, your body will get the benefits of both. Mix up your exercises! It will create variety in your workouts, and your body will benefit with increased strength and endurance from the differences. You will also reduce your risk of overuse injuries by mixing your exercise choices.

Conclusion

There are well-established guidelines for exercise training. Everyone needs a certain amount and frequency of exercise in order to make improvements in physical fitness. However, many different types of exercises fit into those guidelines. If you do the same thing every day, you will no doubt grow tired of it. If you start out walking and find you are avoiding or dreading your exercise, consider the boredom factor. No one says that you have to stay with the same exercise all of the time. Do different things! Turn to page 14 in your *Accountability Journal* to begin establishing the components of a balanced fitness routine.

Also, find exercises that you like to do. Otherwise, it's unlikely that you will stick with a routine. Experiment with different exercises and surprise your body with new and different activities. Also, remember to stay physically active each day. Look for ways to move rather than the easy or most convenient method for performing a task. In doing so, you will continue to push your body to grow stronger and more physically fit each day.

Caloric Considerations

If you are exercising to lose weight, you will be interested in activities that burn calories. On the next page, you will find a list of common exercises and the number of calories expended per hour for two weight groups. Find your weight range and put a check by the activities you are most likely to perform. Remember that the calories expended are measured for an hour.

ENERGY EXPENDITURES

Sedentary	calories		Active
Using Remote Control Device	<1	3	Getting Up to Change Channel
Reclining for 30 Minutes of phone calls	4	20	Standing for 3 10 minute phone calls
Using garage door opener	<1	2-3	Raising garage door 2x/d
Hiring someone to clean and iron	0	152	Ironing and vacuuming each 30 min
Waiting 30 mins for pizza delivery	15	25	Cooking for 30 mins.
Buying presliced vegetables	0	10-13	Washing and slicing vegetables for 15 mins
Using leaf blower for 30 mins	100	150	Raking leaves for 30 mins
Using a lawn service	0	360	Gardening and mowing for 1 h/wk
Using a car wash 1x/month	18	300	Washing and Waxing car, 1h/month
Letting dog out the back door	2	125	Walking dog for 30 mins
Driving 40 mins, walking 5 (parking)	22	60	Walking 15 mins to bus stop 2x/d
Sending e-mail to colleague, 4 min	2-3	6	Walking 1 min, talking (standing) 3 mins
Taking elevator up 3 flights	2-3	15	Walking up 3 flights
Parking as close as possible, 10-s walk	0.3	8	Parking in 1st spot, walking 2 mins, 5x/wk
Letting cashier unload shopping cart	2	6	Unloading full shopping cart
Riding escalator 3x	2	15	Climbing 1 flight of stairs, 3x/wk in mall
Shopping online 1 hour	30	145-240	Shopping at mall, walking 1 hour
Paying at the pump	0.6	5	Walking into station to pay, 1x/wk
Sitting and listening to a lecture, 60 mins	30	70	Giving a lecture

* L. Beil, "What Is Proper Weight? Shake It Up, or Go Figure," *Dallas Morning News,* 30 August 1999, 1F, as adapted in Steven Blair, "The Public Health Problem of Increasing Prevalence Rates of Obesity and What Should Be Done About It," *Mayo Clinic Proceedings* 77.2 (February 2002): 112.

CALORIC EXPENDITURE TABLE

(Average Calories Expended/Hour)

Activity	110-140 lbs	160-190 lbs
Aerobics	290-575	400-800
Baseball	225-255	270-305
Backpacking	290-630	400-800
Basketball	400-690 (Game) 170-515 (Nongame)	560-960 (Game) 240-720 (Nongame)
Bicycling	170-800 (Outdoor) 85-800 (Stationary)	240-1120 (Outdoor) 120-1120 (Stationary)
Bowling	115-170	160-240
Gardening	115-400	160-560
Golf (Walking)	115-400	160-560
Hiking	170-690	240-960
Jogging	460 (12 min/mile) 575 (10 min/mile)	640 (12 min/mile) 800 (10 min/mile)
Racquetball	345-690	480-960
Running	690 (9 min/mile)	960 (9 min/mile)
Skating	230-460	320-640
Stair Climbing	230-460	320-640
Swimming	230-960	320-900
Tennis	230-515	320-720
Walking	115 (30 min/mile) 170 (20 min/mile)	160 (30 min/mile) 240 (20 min/mile)
Weight Training	390-485	530-665

*Health News Network, http://www.healthnewsnet.com/calorie.html

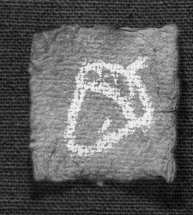

Week Six
Eating Disorders
Kelly Preston

When I was 14 years old, I had one of my most memorable Christmas seasons. For a month I had been a patient in a hospital an hour from my home. My dad and youngest brother picked me up on Christmas morning so that I could be with my family for six hours before going back to the hospital that evening. Although we joyfully celebrated the birth of Christ, the day was also filled with many tears and fears. My family feared for my life because I was a patient in a unit for people struggling with eating disorders and fighting to stay alive.

Thankfully, I am much healthier today than I was on Christmas Day, 1987. My journey has been filled with many ups and downs; however, I praise God for allowing me to struggle with and recover from an eating disorder. This experience has made me who I am today and reminds me daily of my absolute need for Christ.

WHAT ARE EATING DISORDERS?

According to the National Institute of Mental Health *(www.nimh.nih.gov),* eating disorders frequently develop during adolescence or early adulthood. However, some reports indicate their onset during childhood or later in adulthood. The two most common eating disorders are anorexia nervosa and bulimia.

Females are much more likely than males to develop an eating disorder, although the number of males with eating disorders is on the rise. An estimated .5 to 3.7 percent of females suffer from anorexia nervosa in their lifetime, and an estimated 1.1 to 4.2 percent of females suffer from bulimia. While these percentages may seem small, they are, unfortunately, increasing.

Characteristics of Anorexia Nervosa

Anorexia nervosa is characterized by the following:
- intense fear of gaining weight and being fat
- self-starvation
- in females delayed onset or loss of menstrual periods
- distorted body image—thinking one is fat while very thin or emaciated
- obsessive or compulsive exercise

UPREACH

Turn to the "Read the Bible Through" chart on page 95. Locate today's date and read the suggested Scriptures. Follow this plan each day this week.

- isolation from family and friends
- body weight that is 15 percent below normal

Because of severe weight loss, persons with anorexia nervosa can suffer complications such as dry skin and hair, cold hands and feet, weakness, constipation and digestive problems, increased susceptibility to infections and stress fractures, severe electrolyte imbalances, low blood pressure and dizziness, and weakness of the heart muscle that can lead to death. In fact, anorexia nervosa has the highest mortality rate of all mental illnesses.

I can relate to almost all of these characteristics. What began as losing a few pounds from my already petite body turned into a life-consuming obsession. I became so afraid of gaining weight that I counted every calorie and stopped drinking water because it made me feel full. On many occasions I weighed myself at least 25 times per day. If the number on the scale showed any amount of weight gain, I became extremely upset. At a mere 63 pounds, I secretly exercised in my room at night or outdoors by taking our dog for a walk—actually a run.

It wasn't until my senior year of college that I had enough body fat to have a normal menstrual cycle. Although I never fainted, my heart rate and blood pressure were dangerously low. From an emotional perspective, I had no social life because so much of it revolved around food. Instead, I became isolated from friends and family, depressed, and unable to escape from the prison of anorexia nervosa.

Characteristics of Bulimia

The other most common eating disorder is bulimia, characterized by:
- binge-eating (consuming large amounts of food at one sitting while feeling out of control)
- purging (getting rid of food by using laxatives and/or diuretics, self-induced vomiting, and/or compulsive exercise)
- dissatisfaction with one's body
- fear of gaining weight
- mood swings
- isolation from family and friends
- abuse of alcohol or other substances

The binge/purge cycle puts bulimics at high risk for severe complications, including dehydration, weakness, severe electrolyte imbalances, damaged teeth, heart irregularities, digestive and intestinal problems, ruptured esophagus ("food tube"), and death.

Compulsive Exercise

Although I never used laxatives, diuretics, or self-induced vomiting as a means of purging, I did engage in compulsive exercise. I have often termed exercise as my drug of choice. The very act of exercising was a way to escape reality and feelings I didn't want to feel—very much like alcohol does for the alcoholic. If I didn't exercise enough or at all, I would become irritable and anxious. For me, exercise was no longer fun or a way to stay healthy but something I felt like I had to do.

UPREACH

Read 2 Corinthians 10:12-18.

1. How does the apostle Paul characterize these people who compare themselves to each other (v. 12)?

2. Is proper approval found in comparing yourself to another person?
   ❏ yes   ❏ no

3. From whom do we gain ultimate approval (v. 18)?

My friend Lauren agrees. She is a recovering anorexic and bulimic who compulsively exercised as a means of purging. She says, "I experienced severe dehydration and electrolyte imbalances, my menstrual cycle stopped for more than a year, and I isolated myself from all social settings for fear of not being able to control what I did or didn't eat." She was headed down the path of destruction.

According to SCAN (Sports, Cardiovascular and Wellness Nutritionists), a practice group of the American Dietetic Association *(www.nutrifit.org),* "exercise can turn into an unhealthy means of control, and an unrealistic yardstick for measuring self-worth. It becomes a compulsion—a way to avoid life, rather than experience it." Anyone can become addicted to exercise, as evidenced by these characteristics:

- often choosing to exercise beyond the requirements for good health
- stealing time to exercise from work, school, relationships, and social events
- focusing only on the challenge and forgetting that exercise can be fun
- defining self-worth in terms of performance
- rarely or never satisfied with athletic achievements
- unable to savor victory; always pushing on to the next challenge
- justifying excessive behavior by defining oneself as a special elite athlete
- using exercise compulsively to control weight
- experiencing strong feelings of guilt or anxiety if unable to exercise
- not allowing time off to heal injuries
- hiding from emotional pain by working out
- ignoring comments from family and friends about the amount of time engaged in physical activity

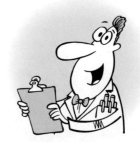

Professor Phitt says:
You may feel you are light years from becoming addicted to exercise! A good rule-of-thumb is 30-45 minutes of exercise 3-5 times per week.

Several physical and psychological consequences can occur from compulsive exercise—stress fractures, dehydration, tendinitis, irregular or absent menstrual cycles in women, anemia, and chronic fatigue syndrome. Depression, anxiety, strained relationships, and social isolation are some psychological and social consequences related to compulsive exercise.

WHAT CAUSES EATING DISORDERS?

What could possibly cause someone to starve oneself and/or binge and purge, even to the point of death? Unfortunately, this question isn't easily answered. Many factors combine to cause eating disorders. Keep in mind that food and weight aren't the real issues but merely the symptoms. What lies beneath—feelings of guilt, fear, low self-esteem, the need for control, and a myriad of other issues—are the real sources of eating disorders.

The following potential causes have been identified by The Center for Eating Disorders *(www.eating-disorders.com):*

- stressful life situations accompanied by a lack of adequate coping skills
- history of trauma (50 percent of bulimics have been sexually abused)
- biological/genetic predisposition
- socio-cultural factors (media and pop-culture messages on weight and appearance)
- family dynamics
- personality traits such as perfectionism, low self-esteem, and depression

Kelley Cousins, a licensed professional counselor with New Life Clinics (*www.newlife.com*) in Birmingham, Alabama, works with individuals who have eating disorders. Ms. Cousins states, "Most individuals with eating disorders don't have a well-established sense of self-identity. Instead, they are too bonded with another person, usually a parent, and not free to be an individual." Therefore, Ms. Cousins suggests that when working with people who have an eating disorder, look at the family of origin.

According to Ms. Cousins, "Once the person's physical being is stabilized, psychological therapy can begin, looking at the underlying, core issues that the person is dealing with. The goal is to build the person's sense of self-worth so that she is able to effectively deal with whatever she is trying to avoid."[1]

The American culture is obsessed with physical appearance. Children are taught at a young age that thin is good and fat is bad. Increasingly, teenage boys experiment with dangerous substances to help them gain muscle and lose fat so they will excel at sports and look good. In essence, we are teaching our children to focus on the outer appearance instead of focusing on someone's heart. Read 1 Samuel 16:1-14 in your Bible. We need to teach our children—and all people, for that matter—that one's worth and value aren't based on how much they weigh or what they look like but on who they are—beautiful, unique creations of our Heavenly Father.

The Slippery Slope

When I was six years old, I started swimming competitively. By the time I was 12, I had joined an elite training team half-an-hour away from my hometown. We swam before school, after school, and twice each day during the summer. When I was 13, I was ranked nationally for my age. Soon after the best meet of my life, I began going down the slippery slope of anorexia nervosa. I quit eating foods with sugar and fat and was barely surviving on 200 calories a day. Within a few months, my weight dropped so drastically that my parents forced me to quit swimming. Before long, I was in the hospital struggling to stay alive.

While it's now clear to me that my eating disorder was a way of coping with feelings of fear, anger, and the need to be in control, I desperately needed help. God's word states that we are to love our neighbor as we love ourselves (Mark 12:31) and that our bodies are a temple of the Holy Spirit (1 Cor. 6:19). I certainly was not loving myself or caring for my body as God's temple. God has done such a work in my life since that time.

TREATMENT FOR EATING DISORDERS

The sooner a person with an eating disorder gets treatment, the more likely she will recover. According to The Eating Disorders Program at The Institute for Living (*www.instituteofliving.com/Eatingdisorders/*), as many as 75 percent of those afflicted with anorexia nervosa or bulimia will recover, while the remaining 25 percent will chronically struggle with the eating disorder. Without treatment, up to 20 percent of people with serious eating disorders die. With treatment, that number falls to 2-3 percent (*Anorexia Nervosa and Related Eating Disorders, Inc., www.anred.com*).

OUTREACH

Encourage someone close to you. Use positive words to build them up and help them to feel valuable.

"If anyone is in Christ, he is a new creation; the old has gone, the new has come."
—2 Corinthians 5:17

People with an eating disorder usually need an interdisciplinary approach to treatment. This may consist of a combination of the following:
- Professional counseling—individual, couples, family, and/or group therapy
- Medical treatment—the use of certain medications prescribed by a physician and/or psychiatrist shown to benefit some persons with eating disorders
- Nutritional counseling—working one-on-one with a registered dietitian who has experience in working with eating disorder clients
- Inpatient hospitalization—used in severe cases of eating disorders, where feeding plans address the person's medical and nutritional needs; in addition, intense psychological therapy takes place

Prior to entering an inpatient treatment center, I saw several psychologists, nutritionists, and medical doctors. Unfortunately, I was so far along in the disease that nothing seemed to help. My parents felt helpless. I finally got to the point of wanting help. My first hospitalization took place in a specialized eating disorders unit. I spent nearly four months re-learning how to eat in a healthy way as well as how to deal with the many struggles going on inside. I met regularly with a psychiatrist, a nutritionist, and a medical doctor. We had group therapy on a variety of topics—everything from body image to learning how to be assertive and how to express our feelings in a healthy manner. As I became physically stable, I learned the role that my feelings, such as anger and fear, have in this complex disease.

Going home was scary because I had the freedom to go back to my old behaviors of not eating and exercising too much—ultimately what happened to me within three years. By 1991, I was back in the hospital, yet the six weeks I was on this adolescent psychiatric unit proved to be invaluable to my understanding of the mind.

God's word says that we have the mind of Christ (1 Cor. 2:16), yet for far too long I had allowed Satan's lies to deceive me. I struggled with Christ being Lord of my life and learned the importance of surrendering each day to Him. God's word says "Choose life" (read Deut. 30:15-20), and I had to choose to stay alive by eating enough healthy food and by learning to exercise for enjoyment and its health benefits.

After leaving the hospital, I immediately started seeing a Christian counselor on a weekly basis, and I continued to see a medical doctor to ensure that my weight remained stable. My doctor put me on a medication for obsessive-compulsive disorders to help minimize these tendencies. I was able to return to swimming and cross-country running, but for the first time in many years, I enjoyed exercising!

During my years in a private Christian college, true healing began. Not only did I become healthier physically and mentally (I was able to stop the medication during this time), but I grew leaps and bounds spiritually. I finally began to take God's word to heart. Part of my recovery has been to allow myself to be loved. My husband has been like Christ to me—loving me unconditionally and encouraging me to be the woman God has called me to be. God is truly amazing!

INREACH
Take time to think about your value in God's eyes. Write three words that describe positive things that God sees in you.

" 'Who has known the mind of the Lord that he may instruct him?' But we have the mind of Christ."
—1 Corinthians 2:16

"We know that in all things God works for the good of those who love him, who have been called according to his purpose."
—Romans 8:28

UPREACH

Read again Psalm 139 in your Bible. Underline verse 14. Consider committing this verse to memory.

Lauren can also testify to God's amazing grace. Thanks to friends who confronted her in loving concern, Lauren sought treatment at Remuda Ranch in Wickenburg, Arizona *(www.remuda-ranch.com)*. She spent 45 days there re-learning how to eat and searching within. "It was exhausting to search my soul because for so long I had denied how I felt. Starving myself or binging and purging was how I coped, and now I had to learn how to cope with life in healthy ways. It's about replacing lies with God's truth because the mind is a battlefield." After returning home, Lauren struggled to maintain her healthy coping mechanisms, often resorting to binging and purging. But with the help of outpatient therapy, medication, and support from friends, she is continuing to move forward in her recovery process.[2]

Helping a person recognize who they are in Christ is important because individuals with eating disorders usually have low self-esteem. Hopefully over time and by the grace of God, they will see themselves as Christ does—fearfully and wonderfully made (Ps. 139:14). Abundant life (John 10:10) exists beyond eating disorders!

The following self-tests will help you determine if you tend toward an eating or compulsive exercise disorder, or if you have a friend or loved one with these symptoms. Circle *yes* or *no* and then total your score for each test.

SELF-TESTS

How can I determine if I have an eating disorder?[3]
1. I worry about gaining weight. Yes No
2. I am preoccupied with losing weight. Yes No
3. I frequently diet or feel the need to be on a diet. Yes No
4. My mood depends on my weight (for example, if I gain one pound I am depressed, irritable, and so on). Yes No
5. I feel bad about myself if I gain weight. Yes No
6. If I gain one pound, I worry that I will continue to gain weight. Yes No
7. I think of certain foods as being either good or bad and feel guilty about eating bad foods. Yes No
8. I use food to comfort myself. Yes No
9. At times when I am eating, I feel I have lost control. Yes No
10. I spend lots of time thinking about food and when I will eat. Yes No
11. I try to hide how much I eat. Yes No
12. I have thought about (or have) self-induced vomiting as a means of weight control. Yes No
13. After eating, I may use laxatives, diuretics, exercise, and other ways to prevent weight gain. Yes No
14. I am dissatisfied with my body size and shape. Yes No
15. I eat until I feel stuffed. Yes No

If you answered yes to five or more questions, you may have an eating disorder.

How can you recognize whether or not someone you care about has an eating disorder?[4]

1. You've noticed a weight change unrelated to a medical condition. Yes No
2. You've noticed a preoccupation with food. Yes No
3. You've noticed a preoccupation with weight. Yes No
4. You've noticed a preoccupation with appearance. Yes No
5. You've noticed compulsive or excessive exercise. Yes No
6. You've noticed abnormal eating habits such as severe diet, cutting up food in tiny pieces, or playing with food. Yes No
7. You've noticed large amounts of food purchases disappear quickly. Yes No
8. You've noticed increased social isolation and/or depression. Yes No
9. You've heard dissatisfaction with weight despite excessive weight loss. Yes No
10. You've noticed frequent trips to the restroom, especially after meals. Yes No
11. You've noticed the smell of vomit in the restroom. Yes No
12. You've noticed frequent dieting despite excessive weight loss. Yes No

Yes to four or more questions should cause concern.

How do you know if you have a problem with compulsive exercise?[5]

1. Do you find that you regularly adjust your exercise according to how much you ate earlier or on the preceding day? Yes No
2. Are you concerned to terrified about being overweight? Yes No
3. Did your interest in exercise begin with a desire to lose weight? Yes No
4. Do you fear not exercising each day because you think you'll gain weight? Yes No
5. Are you preoccupied with food and calories and calculate what you are allowed to eat each day according to how much time you can give to exercise? Yes No
6. Have you gone on eating binges where you feel you cann't stop? Yes No
7. Do you exercise an excessive amount after a binge? Yes No
8. Are you preoccupied with being thinner and having a lower body mass/lean muscle ratio like elite athletes? Yes No
9. Do you think about burning calories as you exercise? Yes No
10. Do you ever vomit, take laxatives, or diuretics after a meal or binge to feel thinner or to attempt to lose calories? Yes No
11. Do you feel virtuous when restricting your food intake or exercising? Yes No
12. Do others tell you that you exercise too much? Yes No

If you answered yes to six or more of these questions, your exercise may be based on an eating disorder.

GETTING HELP FOR YOURSELF

Perhaps you realized that you may be struggling with an eating disorder. Or, you may know you have an eating disorder but are afraid to tell anyone or to get help. Recall that eating disorders are very serious problems that can be deadly. Your Heavenly Father doesn't want you to be imprisoned by an eating disorder any longer. There's hope in Him! The following tips are important for you to consider:

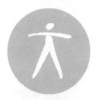

OUTREACH

If you identify a person with a possible eating disorder, read carefully the topic, "Helping a Person with an Eating Disorder," on page 56.

INREACH

Admitting a problem is the most difficult yet most important step in healing. If you recognize in yourself certain behaviors that cause you concern, will you pray about seeking help?

❏ Yes   ❏ No

• Admit to yourself that you have an eating disorder. This is the first and often the most difficult step in the recovery process.
• Seek professional help. Many counselors and even Christian treatment centers help people with eating disorders.
• Confide in someone you trust for support and encouragement. Having the support of a friend or family member helps as you walk through this journey.
• Remember that recovery is a long road, and there is no quick fix for your eating disorder. Professional help and support from loved ones makes the road to recovery much easier.
• Pray for God to renew your mind (Rom. 12:2) so that you will know what a wonderful creation you are, that you are completely loved as you are (read Eph. 3:14-21), and that you are at your loveliest when you strive for the beauty that lasts (read 1 Pet. 3:3-10).

HELPING A PERSON WITH AN EATING DISORDER

When helping persons with eating disorders, family members, friends, and even health care professionals may become discouraged and feel helpless. Because of the complexity of these disorders, no magic bullet or quick cure exists. However, you can encourage and support people with eating disorders.

Recognize the power of an eating disorder. These disorders have a life of their own, overpowering a person's logic and will. Therefore, he or she must come to the point of wanting to change and wanting help. Suggest professional help and various resources, but realize that recovery is his or her responsibility, not yours.[6]

Be compassionate toward the individual. Logic doesn't work, but love does. It's easy to focus on food and weight—even argue about such things—but these are only symptoms of a serious, deeper problem. Focus on how the individual is feeling—scared, out of control, guilty, and so on. Ask the person how you can help. Listening can be the most important thing you can do.

Know your limits. Most people with eating disorders need professional help, so referral to a counselor is often necessary. Pray for God's healing in the person's life. **He is able!** For more information on how to help someone you care about with an eating disorder, visit *www.mirror-mirror.org/approve.htm*.

[1]Personal interview, February 2002.
[2]Personal interview, February 2002.
[3]Adapted from "Do You Have an Eating Disorder?" <*http://www.eating-disorders.com/doyouqz.htm*> (21 March 2001).
[4]Adapted from "How Can I Recognize if Someone I Care About Has an Eating Disorder?" <*http://www.eating-disorders.com/doessome.htm*> (21 March 2002).
[5]Adapted from Rebecca Prussin, Phillip Harvey, and Theresa Foy DiGeronimo, *Hooked on Exercise: How to Understand and Manage Exercise Addiction* (New York: Simon & Schuster, 1992), as quoted in Sherry Fixelle, "What is Compulsive Exercise?" <*http://www.nutrifit.org/nutr_info/compulsiveex.html#know*> (19 July 2002).
[6]If the person with an eating disorder is younger than 18 years of age, parents have a legal and moral responsibility to get their child professional help. If the person with an eating disorder is older than 18 years of age, he or she is legally an adult and can refuse treatment if he or she isn't ready to change.

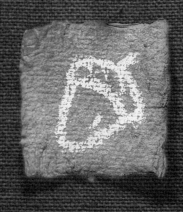

Week Seven
Managing Stress
Susan Lanford

I love to write! In recent years God has used my writing assignments to focus my attention on important issues in my life. It's happened often enough that the call to produce a chapter on managing stress should have given me pause. But it's a subject that fascinates me and one I've enjoyed studying and teaching for several years. I concluded I was safe from any object lessons if I tackled this one.

In the precise week I had set aside to complete it, I became very ill. I learned I had mononucleosis ("Look at it this way, Mom," said my college-aged daughter, "you caught a young person's disease!"), bronchitis, and pneumonia. I've logged seven trips to the doctor's office, numerous prescriptions, one breathing treatment, two steroid shots, one x-ray, three blood draws, three weeks of missed work, and enough time on the couch to make me physically ill again when I walk into that room. The weakness, coughing, and lethargy persists 10 weeks later, but I know I will recover at some point in the future.

This stretch of illness began two weeks after Christmas, which included 1800 miles of travel. The month before Christmas an unexpected work project required long hours into several nights. The five months before Christmas I started a new teaching job. The adjustments needed to get up to speed meant many extra hours on a consistent basis.

So why did I get sick? Surely the viral elements explain much of it. Just as surely the accumulation of months of overwork contributed to a weakened immune system where the viral Vikings gained a beachhead and won the day. Humbly, I confess to God that I've learned another valuable life lesson—that feeling fulfilled, challenged, and happy while overworking still leaves me vulnerable to the effects of stress. In my chastened frame of mind then, let's talk stress!

HOW DID WE GET SO STRESSED?
Some think stress is a convenient cop-out invented in the last 40 years to provide a reason for underachievement, overcommitment, and moodiness! Truth is, the physiological phenomenon known as the stress response is imbedded in us down

to the cellular level and has existed since our earliest days on earth. It is the body going on point, into high gear, at warp speed—use any popular term you'd like. It's the automatic, instinctive response that makes us jerk our hand off a hot burner, jump back on the curb at the sound of tires screeching, or lift a heavy object off its trapped victim. Our earliest ancestors bested woolly mammoths and evaded marauding tribes because of this instinctive energy surge, and we possess the same physiological instincts today. Read Luke 12:22-31 in your Bible.

Over four millennia ago, Chinese sages observed that illness followed frustration, and the Egyptians were prescribed to display cheerfulness and optimism for their good health. Greek physicians ordered rest and relaxation to promote healing from illness. The Bible's wisdom literature asserts: "A cheerful heart is good medicine, but a broken spirit saps a person's strength" (Prov. 17:22, NLT).

Fast forward to the turn of the last century: the pioneering medical researcher, Dr. Walter Cannon of Harvard Medical School, coined the familiar phrase "fight or flight response" to describe the physiology of being threatened—a key word in the definition of stress. Move on to the 1950s when the name most associated with understanding stress emerged—Dr. Hans Selye. The first to use the word *stress* to mean the body's response to any pressure or demand, he is also credited with resurrecting the ancient notions that disease could result from the failure to adapt to stressful conditions. In other words, Dr. Selye was interested in what is known as stressors—and in how we adapt to those stressors, the stress response.

Then, in the late 1960s, Dr. Herbert Benson of Harvard Medical School, along with Doctors Robert Keith Wallace and Archie F. Wilson at the University of California-Irvine, discovered that learned relaxation techniques could slow metabolism and counteract the intensity of the body's stress response. Dr. Benson termed this "the relaxation response," a key component in stress management.

Since that time, the evidence has accumulated to staggering proportions: Stress is a major correlate, if not a cause, in most medical diagnoses and chronic conditions today. Studies indicate that 75-90 percent of visits to primary care physicians are made by the chronically anxious or the worried well. In other words, the accumulated effects of stress over time weaken our immune systems and begin to break down the body's major organ systems. It makes us sick!

For example, one of the earliest links established between stress and disease involved heart disease. Years ago, physicians warned Type A patients to act against type to lessen the stress in their lives or risk coronary attacks or disease. Research now indicates that the risk isn't so much in their overwork, ambition, or drive, and thankfully so, because we need the Type A people of the world. The risk is in being chronically bitter, chronically angry, and chronically cynical, which weakens heart muscles and makes such folks so vulnerable. Data from such different groups as bereaved spouses, caregivers of the long-term ill, and the unhappily married also confirm that their immune functioning was more compromised than people of similar demographics but without such difficult, emotional stressors.

"Stress is the spice of life … complete freedom from stress is death."
—Hans Selye

Words to Know

Stress—the body's response to any pressure, demand, or change.

Stressor—the stimulus or event that prompts the body's stress response. Stressors can be internal (thoughts, beliefs) and external (circumstances, relationships).

Relaxation Response—the learned behaviors which give needed rest and recuperation to our minds and bodies to help undo the negative, wearing effects of stress. Example: breathing techniques.

Half of work-related issues—absenteeism, reduced loyalty to employers, poor product quality, underproductivity, and rising insurance claims—are now considered stress-based phenomena. Offering stress management options has become a premium human resource task in today's corporate world.

Medical researchers now believe that the spiritual discipline of forgiveness actually lessens stress on the body and promotes health. Researchers at the University of Tennessee found higher blood pressure in subjects who were unforgiving. Subjects in a Hope College (Michigan) study were asked to remember past grievances against them. In doing so, they registered higher blood pressure, increased heart rates, and greater muscle tension. The Forgiveness Project at Stanford University has documented harmful physical effects of mismanaged anger and hostility.

AND HOW DID YOU GET SO STRESSED?

That's easy—you're alive! The only stress-free life is the life-free life. But not all stress is bad. Dr. Selye divided stress into eustress, or good stress, and distress, or bad stress. Eustress motivates you to set and reach goals, initiate changes, solve problems, and take on big tasks. Research shows that increasing stress is positively linked with increasing performance and efficiency—up to a point. But when stress has no relief—even eustress—the body and mind wear down, resulting in distress.

Notice the diagram below. Reaching the apex of the curve means if the stress persists, then performance and efficiency decrease. You've had those times when it takes much longer to complete—or even start—a task that used to be routine, when you're working harder with less efficiency or fewer results.

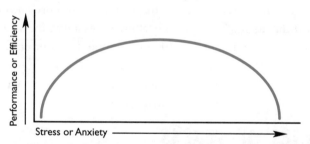

Here's what happens when your body responds to both types of stress.
1. You perceive a threat and physiologically you go on full alert.
2. Your limbic system kicks in and releases various chemicals into your body:
   Adrenaline—Making nutrients available to the body for strenuous action.
   Noradrenaline—Increasing blood pressure and blood flow to the muscles.
   Glucocorticoids—Making fat available for energy, increasing blood flow, and increasing alertness in the brain.
3. Your pupils dilate, giving you clearer vision; your breathing increases, giving your body more oxygen to burn the added fuel; you can now act with more strength and speed.
4. You become more vigilant, sharply focused, and forget everything else you were thinking about as your brain's dopamine system changes the neurochemical balances in your brain.
5. Your brain has you focused and prepared to fight or flee the danger.

"Then Peter came to Jesus and asked, 'Lord, how many times shall I forgive my brother when he sins against me? Up to seven times?' Jesus answered, 'I tell you, not seven times, but seventy-seven times.' "
—Matthew 18:21-22

Words to Know

Distress—bad stress; the sense that life is unmanageable which negatively affects our bodies, minds, and spirit.

Eustress—good stress; positive life changes or circumstances to which we easily adapt.

Stress response—the automatic response of the body which elevates heart rate, blood pressure, blood sugar, makes the breathing shallow and quick, and floods the extremities with a chemical boost to meet a threat or flee from a threat (fight or flight response).

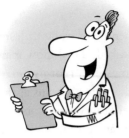

Professor Phitt says:
Physical exercise is a known stress-reducer. Heed these words, written by a wise man many years ago:

"Those who think they have not time for bodily exercise will sooner or later have to find time for illness."
—Edward Stanley,
15th Earl of Derby

INREACH
Select one of your daily stressors. Assign it to one of these categories. Then list ways you can reduce or modify this stressor.

These responses are normal and critically important if you are to cope with stressors. Animals with their adrenal glands removed are likely to die under stress. Humans without adrenal glands must take glucocorticoid supplements to cope physically. The stress response is a healthy part of human psychophysiology.

Over time, however, the accumulated effects of being kicked into high gear over and over wear us out. These effects include:
- increased blood pressure which can lead to stroke and heart attacks;
- increased blood cholesterol levels;
- damage to muscle tissue;
- steroid diabetes;
- infertility;
- inhibition of the inflammatory responses which makes it more difficult for the body to heal itself after injury;
- suppression of the immune system which makes one more susceptible to infection, parasites, environmental pollutants, and even cancer.

Two key truths need your full attention as we summarize:
1. Your body cannot distinguish between its stressors. It initiates the full alert stress response anytime it perceives a threat, whether it is physical (an attacker), emotional (hearing sad news), cognitive (believing you won't meet a deadline), spiritual (doubts about God's presence when you suffer), behavioral (shouting at your family), or relational (loss of a spouse). This stress response, which helps insure our physical safety, actually hurts us physically when it activates for all these other sorts of threats.
2. The body needs time to recover from this response. In more ancient times when physical threats might occur only a few times a day, the stress response provided protection for the body without harming it. In our culture, the typical adult experiences 40-80 stress responses a day, producing tremendous wear and tear on the body and allowing no possibility of recovery between episodes. For these two reasons alone, we need to manage stress.

CATEGORIES OF STRESS
The following statements are helpful for understanding life's stress. You have …
- stress you can avoid and stress you can't avoid;
- stress you can modify;
- stress to which you contribute or which you create for yourself.

Read the list again and find the repeating pronoun. See it? Yes; it's *you!* You have stress—or stressors—you can avoid or modify. For example, you arrive home most evenings tied in knots because of rush-hour traffic. Because of the frustration, you are short-tempered with your family, unmotivated to tackle tasks at home, and sleeping fitfully each night. What are your choices?
- Avoid this stress: rearrange work hours to miss the worst of rush hour.
- Move closer to work, find alternate routes, carpool, or use commuter transit.
- Switch from listening to news of the day's horrors or talk radio tantrums to stations or tapes of calming words or music.

Just don't passively act as though you have no choices and continue inflicting damage on you and those around you because you're stressed!

In addition to stress you can modify, you have stressors of your own doing, stress you create or to which you contribute. Again, this puts the power of choice back in your hands; different behaviors and healthier thoughts will lessen your stress. Here an example: You agree to decorate 20 tables for a fund-raising dinner using items from past events in order to save money. But you feel compelled to show up the decorating of previous years. So, you order rare, stunning tropical flowers, paying out of your pocket, and get a notice that your account is overdrawn. That's stress to which you contribute. Staying with the original plan lessens the stress.

You have stress you cannot avoid—that too is life! Even so, your choices about how you respond make all the difference. For example, the day after the the birth of your wonderful child, you suddenly recall horror tales of something called the terrible twos. For the next two years, you obsess about how awful life will be then. Or, you smile and think, I have two years to read about toddlers, talk to other parents, prepare myself and the house—and I believe I'll live to tell about it!

It's not as ridiculous an example as you might think. Normal people experience this paralysis about the next steps in life—planning a wedding, choosing a college, approaching mid-life, raising a teenager—and then act as though they were completely caught off-guard and have lived through an utterly unique experience.

Stress is yet another way we learn just how complex we are. But you cannot praise God because you are "fearfully and wonderfully made" (Ps. 139:14) and live your life as if your daily choices don't matter. The Psalmist, so articulate about the joys and pains of life, certainly knew this when he wrote Psalm 31. Read the verses in the margin. Underline the stress symptoms.

Tell the truth about it.

Take note of the clues your body, mind, and spirit give you. Initially, you may feel worse admitting to your stress. But stop labeling your life as hectic, busy, overworked, pressure-packed, and so forth. In other words, tell the truth about your life! Unfortunately, busyness is a badge of honor in this culture. We play an ongoing game of "Top that!" and if we win the game, we're rewarded with the sounds of sympathetic groans. Then we know we've earned our martyr status and their respect for all we handle.

STRESS WARNING SIGNALS

I once worked in a hospital-based stress management program. Our participants came for many reasons, but typically half of each group were there because their physicians prescribed it to improve their health. Almost without exception, those participants came to registration mumbling about their doctors, insisting they weren't stressed, and feeling they were going to waste their time in this class. We would begin by handing them the "Stress Warning Signals" self-test on page 62.[1]

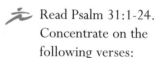 Read Psalm 31:1-24. Concentrate on the following verses:

"I am in distress;
    my eyes grow weak
       with sorrow,
    my soul and my body
       with grief.
My life is consumed
       by anguish
    and my years by groaning;
my strength fails because
       of my affliction,
    and my bones grow weak.
I have become like
       broken pottery."
       —Psalm 31:9-10,12

Mark this list with 1 = seldom or never, 2 = sometimes, or 3 = frequently. If you're pressed for time, mark only your 3's, your frequent symptoms. Frequent means whatever you say it means.

STRESS WARNING SIGNALS

1 = Seldom or Never   2 = Sometimes   3 = Frequently

Physical Symptoms

____ Headaches	____ Back pain	____ Weariness
____ Indigestion	____ Tight neck and shoulders	____ Ringing in ears
____ Stomachaches	____ Racing heart	____ Dizziness
____ Sweaty palms	____ Restlessness	____ Difficulty sleeping

Behavioral Symptoms

____ Excess smoking	____ Grinding teeth while asleep	____ Bossiness
____ Overuse of alcohol	____ Compulsive gum chewing	____ Compulsive eating
____ Critical of others	____ Unable to get things done	

Emotional Symptoms

____ Crying	____ Nervousness	____ Feeling lonely
____ Anger	____ Edginess: ready to explode	____ Anxiety
____ Easily upset	____ Feeling powerless	____ Boredom (no
____ Unhappy for no reason	____ Overwhelming sense of pressure	meaning to things)

Cognitive Symptoms

____ Forgetfulness	____ Trouble thinking clearly	____ Lack of creativity
____ Constant worry	____ Thoughts of running away	____ Loss of sense of
____ Memory loss	____ Inability to make decisions	humor

Relational Symptoms

____ Isolation	____ Clamming up	____ Intolerance
____ Resentment	____ Nagging	____ Often alone
____ Distrust	____ Hiding out	____ Lack of intimacy
____ Using people	____ Fewer contacts with friends	____ Lashing out verbally/physically

Spiritual Symptoms

____ Emptiness	____ Looking for magic	____ Loss of meaning
____ Loss of direction	____ Doubt	____ Cynicism
____ Unforgiveness	____ Insistence on control	____ Apathy
____ Martyrdom	____ Complete lack of control	

UPREACH

If you identified one or more spiritual symptoms, would a daily quiet time help you manage these symptoms?
❏ Yes   ❏ No

If you don't have a daily quiet time, begin today by spending five minutes alone with God. Then, increase the number of minutes over time.

Care about stress and you.

If you begin telling yourself the truth about the effects of stress in your life, you'll also acknowledge that frequent headaches are not OK; chronic lethargy isn't acceptable; repeatedly alienating those with whom you live and work isn't the proof of success. With all that in mind, let me suggest some responses to what you see when you look at your stress self-test.

First, get up-to-date on medical checkups. Any symptom occurring frequently needs your attention. It's possible your daily stomachache is an ulcer, your frequent memory loss is depression, or your teeth-grinding will only stop when you wear a dental appliance at night.

Now, look only at your 3's, one at a time, and dedicate yourself to answering these investigative questions:
1. Who am I with when this symptom occurs?
2. When does this symptom occur?
3. What else is happening when I'm aware of this symptom?
4. Where am I when I feel this way?
5. Why does (or doesn't) it bother me that I frequently experience this symptom?

Soon, you'll gain enough insight into the source of your symptom that you can begin modifying the stressor or changing your response to it—and the symptom will become less frequent. This process only works, though, if you are willing to lose the game of who's most important because they are the busiest! Implement healthy changes into your life that enable you to better manage stress. In fact, effective stress management is effective life management. The remainder of this chapter along with all the *Fit 4* programs will get you there.

Take this self-test three or four times a year to see how well or how poorly you're adapting to current life challenges. When I begin managing stress instead of allowing it to manage me, the differences are reflected in my answers. The 3's reduce to 2's or 1's; some disappear altogether!

A CHANGE OF MIND CAN CHANGE YOUR LIFE

Stress, like religion and taxes, is very personal. What stresses you won't bother me. We perceive the same events or circumstances differently. Perceptions are very potent. If we believe we are incapable or inadequate when threatened, then most likely our responses will reflect that feeling, which in turn becomes another stressor needing our attention and sapping our strength. Hence, the title of this section is your greatest stress management ploy: realize that a change of mind—of beliefs and thoughts—can change your life.

A helpful model for recognizing the power of our thoughts is called cognitive distortions—patterns of thinking that are stress-producing. You'll see a list on page 101. Read them over carefully; anyone can find at least one personal tendency on that list—and if we are honest, we'll find several!

OUTREACH

You may have identified a stressful person in your life! Check ways you can deal more effectively with this individual so that your stress level will be reduced:

❑ avoid encounters
❑ refuse to take comments personally
❑ use humor to deflect his or her remarks
❑ place less importance on his or her opinions
❑ pray more about this relationship; ask God to bless this person
❑ other?_____

"Summing it all up, friends, I'd say you'll do best by filling your minds and meditation on things true, noble, reputable, authentic, compelling, gracious—the best, not the worst; the beautiful, not the ugly; things to praise, not things to curse. Put into practice what you learned from me, what you heard and saw and realized. Do that, and God, who makes everything work together, will work you into his most excellent harmonies."
—Philippians 4:8-9,
The Message

Unspoken assumptions—"This always happens to me!" and "If it can go bad, it will happen to me!"—can turn an inconvenient situation into a personal crisis. Challenge your assumptions. In addition, humor is another helpful tool—recognizing the general absurdity of much of our everyday lives.

The rest of Paul's paragraph to the Philippians is so fitting. Read how he encouraged these believers to think in Philippians 4:8-9.

Change Your Mind About These Things

Read the verses in parentheses in each of the following statements. Underline the truth in your Bible.

1. Decide to live in a big world. Jesus taught us to pray for God's kingdom to come. Caring about God's activity in the world protects you from despair when something in your world crumbles because you know the perfect peace God gives to those whose minds stay on Him and trust Him (Isa. 26:3).

2. Notice when your life is confusing or cluttered. "God is not a God of disorder but of peace" (1 Cor. 14:33).

3. Think before acting, especially speaking! "Reckless words pierce like a sword, but the tongue of the wise brings healing" (Prov. 12:18).

4. Value God's creative design in everyone; treat others as if they matter. "If it is possible, as far as it depends on you, live at peace with everyone" (Rom. 12:18).

5. Embrace a simple, quiet life (1 Thess. 4:11). Put enough stillness, silence, and reflection in your life that you will recognize God's voice (remember young Samuel?) and imitate Jesus (see Phil. 2:1-8). This choice relieves you of excessive worry over what others think of you or how they judge you. Reread Matthew 6, and you'll hear Jesus say three times, " 'Do not worry.' " He implied that anxiety is within our control.

6. Believe in the God who made you from dirt (Gen. 2:7) and declared you a little lower than the angels (Ps. 8:5), who knows you intimately (Ps. 139:1-16) and loves you unconditionally (Rom. 5:6-8), who suffered horribly (Isa. 53:3-5) so that you and I could live abundantly (John 10:10), who made plans for us to have hope and a future (Jer. 29:11), a life beyond anything we could ask or imagine. And in Him, find your rest (Matt. 11:28-29).

---

[1]Adapted from Herbert Benson, M.D. and Eileen M. Stuart, R.N., M.S. *The Wellness Book: The Comprehensive Guide to Maintaining Health and Treating Stress-Related Illness* (New York: Simon and Shuster, 1993), 182.

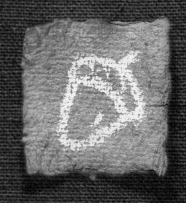

Week Eight
Successful Aging
Michael Parker and George F. Fuller

As advocates of successful aging, medical professionals who serve in the field of geriatrics focus on ways to help seniors avoid disease and disability, maximize their cognitive and physical fitness, remain actively engaged in life, and adopt an attitude of life-long learning and spiritual growth. Despite their efforts, geriatric professionals are often confronted by the reality that many of the discoveries about aging successfully are ignored. For example, some seniors won't take their medications; others refuse to change their eating or exercise habits. As a result, many older persons suffer from diabetes, depression, heart disease, stroke, and other problems that could be delayed, prevented, or treated successfully.

Part of the problem is that many seniors, their families, and even the church are poorly informed about the truths of aging in America. This preoccupation with negative, often false, stereotypes of aging has overshadowed the major importance of lifestyle in maintaining health and vigor.

Rowe and Kahn, two leading researchers in the field of aging, developed a model for successful aging that summarized decades of research. Before highlighting their model and an important addition to it, let's turn our attention to false beliefs or myths about the aging process. Aging myths that operate in our society as partial truths are, to a large degree, false. We will review several of the most frequently circulated myths—single sentence assertions that have some link with reality but are in fundamental conflict with the latest research findings.[1] Myths about aging must be replaced with the truths revealed in the Bible and modern science.

MYTH I: TO BE OLD IS TO BE SICK.
Dr. Robert Butler, the first director of a department of geriatric medicine and the founding director of the National Institute on Aging, was the first to employ the term *ageism* in his Pulitzer Prize-winning book *Why Survive?: Being Old in America.* He described ageism as a form of prejudice in which older persons are viewed as sick, demented, frail, disabled, powerless, sexless, passive, alone, or unable to learn.[2] In describing the seniors in his church, one pastor commented,

UPREACH

How are these biblical characters models for successful aging?

Elizabeth–Luke 1:5-7,24-25

Simeon–Luke 2:25-32

Anna–Luke 2:36-38

"I have fast go's, slow go's, and no go's." When these negative stereotypes were challenged, he realized that the "no go's" did, indeed, "go;" they provided needed leadership and ministry through prayer and other means.

This pastor's initial views of some of his senior members were neither biblical nor scientifically accurate. Experts in aging have played a part in stereotyping the aging person, as well, by focusing on late life disease and disability. The truth is that most older people are experiencing less disability than ever before, reporting higher levels of health than during earlier seasons of our history, and, in general, are experiencing the highest levels of health and sustained periods of independence in our nation's history.

Most elderly people today suffer from what geriatricians call chronic, long-term disease (like arthritis, diabetes, hypertension and heart disease, vision and hearing problems). However, leading experts in aging report major reductions in the prevalence of three key forerunners to chronic disease: high blood pressure, high cholesterol levels, and smoking. Furthermore, major reductions in the incidence of arthritis, hardening of the arteries (arteriosclerosis), hypertension, stroke, and lung disease (emphysema) occurred between 1982 and 1989. Dental health has also improved significantly.

Two older persons of the same age and with the same medical conditions (disease) can function at entirely different levels … one might be a Supreme Court Justice, while the other might be a frail, dependent nursing home resident. The reason for the difference in their functioning levels is what experts call functional status, the capacity of a person to live and function without assistance. Experts assess a person's functional capacities using two methods: instrumental activities of daily living (IDALs, for example, the ability to cook for himself/herself, manage finances) and activities of daily living (ADLs, for example, feeding, bathing, toileting). What does research suggest about how seniors do in these critical areas?

One indication of how seniors function is suggested in the percentage of older persons who live in nursing homes. The percentage of individuals over 65 living in nursing homes continues to decline. Currently less than 5 percent reside in these institutions, down from 6.3 percent in 1982. Another indication is how they describe their own health status. Surveys suggest that most seniors describe themselves as being free of disability. Research indicates that of those aged 65 to 74 in 1994, a full 89 percent reported no disability whatsoever.

While the proportion of elderly who are fully functioning and robust does decline with advancing age, almost 75 percent of seniors between the ages of 75 to 84 reported no disability. Rather than becoming more dependent, one theory (the Compression Morbidity theory) maintains that the percentage of seniors experiencing an active life and delayed disease and disability will continue to increase. Even among the oldest (85 and older), the majority of elderly live independently with little disability. In summarizing decades of research, Rowe and Kahn debunk the myth that to be old is to be sick: "We are delighted to observe increasing momentum toward the emergence of a physically and cognitively fit, nondisabled, active elderly population. The combination of longer life and less illness is adding life to years as well as years to life."[3]

MYTH 2: YOU CAN'T TEACH AN OLD DOG NEW TRICKS.

This myth refers to the inability of older persons to remain life-long learners. This myth is perpetuated in the negative attitudes among many older persons about learning to use the computer and the Internet. Research suggests that though seniors may require a slower pace to learn new information, they can learn new information and may be able to act upon new learning more effectively than younger persons. Older people can place new learning within their context of extensive experience. Organizational research suggests that seniors have an innovative advantage over youth with newly acquired information because their experience compensates for or even goes beyond the flexibility of youth.

When it comes to learning, society is age-graded. Most systems are designed for the young and operate as if there were three distinct periods of life: education, work, and retirement. As a result, many of our institutions of learning (for example, schools, and churches) don't take into consideration the slower rate necessary for optimum learning to occur with seniors. Most churches support age-graded Sunday School classes, yet the biblical model suggests that the old should teach the young (Ps. 71). Our churches need to cultivate attitudes and programs that foster an attitude of life-long learning and provide opportunities for seniors to instruct and teach the young. During pre-Desert Storm deployment, the only senior in the Heidelberg, Germany chapel provided a tremendous, calming influence. As many of us prepared for war, this dear senior, a veteran of World War II, helped American soldiers facing uncertainties in battle to focus on the sovereignty of God and gain peace and assurance for the duties that lay before them.

Research suggests that the majority of elderly show little to no mental decline. In one study, those aged 74-81 showed no mental decline over a seven-year period.[4] Though dementia, particularly Alzheimer's disease, is ever present, many fears about memory loss are exaggerated. The reaction times of youth are generally superior to seniors, but older persons have shown significant and permanent improvements with training in cognitive reasoning (for example, practice games that enhance memory), inductive reasoning, and spatial orientation. The keys to late life learning are:
- to develop a learning climate that allows seniors to work at their own pace;
- to provide opportunities to practice newly acquired skills;
- to monitor the rate of learning so that seniors aren't placed in situations of comparison with younger learners.[5]

Though dementia has no cure, exercise, maintenance of a strong support system, and an attitude of confidence in managing problems, coupled with the acquisition of memory-enhancement techniques, can greatly increase a senior's capacity to maintain cognitive function and to learn. In summary, research suggests that the

INREACH
Describe how you plan to spend your senior years. Do any of your plans include continuing education?

elders can sharpen their intellectual capacities and avoid the cycle of mental insufficiency stemming from inactivity.

MYTH 3: THE HORSE IS OUT OF THE BARN.

This myth would have you believe that it is too late to reduce the risk of disease and disability. It suggests that if you have been smoking, not exercising, drinking too much, or overeating fatty foods for most of your life, it is too late to change. Fortunately, research affirms that lost function can be recovered and that the risk of disease and disability can be reduced. In some cases, the level of functioning (for example, exercise) can be increased by beginning healthy habits early and sustaining them throughout life. Good, old-fashioned clean living seems to work best.

Seniors who lose excessive weight, stop smoking, and begin to exercise experience significant health changes through a reduced incidence of disease and disability. For example, when the weight drops for certain categories of older people, they reduce their risk for heart disease. Dietary changes (more grains and vegetables) can result in lower blood pressure levels for certain older persons. Some must take medication, but many older persons resist this counsel because of their age. Yet, the pharmaceutical treatment of certain forms of hypertension has reduced strokes in older men by ⅓ and heart attacks by more than ¼.[6]

Though with age the body loses physical function, many reductions in physical performance are reversible. Exercise can increase physical fitness, increase muscle size and strength, favorably influence balance, and help prevent falls. Lifting weights and other forms of resistance training can develop bone strength and density, limit the effects of diseases like osteoporosis, and help improve balance, as well. So, don't believe this myth! Remember, it is never too late to begin a healthy lifestyle change!

MYTH 4: THE SECRET TO SUCCESSFUL AGING IS TO CHOOSE YOUR PARENTS WISELY.

Though one's genetic inheritance and ability to age well are related, most of the variance in understanding the aging process is associated with lifestyle. This good news means that older people can make choices that help determine their health-related futures. Diet, exercise, and even medications may delay, or completely eliminate, the development of certain diseases. The longevity found in many families can be related to similar lifestyle features (eating, exercise habits).

Heredity's strongest influence appears to be in the development of genetic diseases that can shorten life (some cancers). As we grow older, the influence of genetics becomes less important, and lifestyle becomes more important. The degree to which one is filled with vitality and actively engaged in life is primarily related to non-genetic factors.

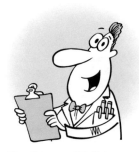

Professor Phitt says:
What lifestyle change(s) have you made as a result of *Fit 4?*

Remember to record your progress in your *Accoutability Journal.*

MYTH 5: THE LIGHTS MAY BE ON, BUT THE VOLTAGE IS LOW.

This myth implies that older people are sexless, or at least uninterested in sex. When partners are available, sexuality in late life is neither rare nor inappropriate. In general, sexual activity does decrease with age, but major individual differences occur among the elderly. Chronological age isn't the key factor. Physiological changes (decline in testosterone) and certain health conditions (like diabetes, heart disease, and hypertension) can impede sexual function, especially in men.

Rowe and Kahn describe a study that found that at age 68, about 70 percent of men were sexually active on a regular basis, but by age 78, the percentage of sexually active men dropped significantly. Overall health and the availability of a partner are factors that influence sexual activity. A distinction needs to be made between forms of physical intimacy and sexual intercourse: "The voltage is never too low" for affectionate physical contact. Such contact "may help keep the lights on."[7]

MYTH 6: THE ELDERLY DON'T PULL THEIR OWN WEIGHT.

The last myth may be the most damaging of all in that it implies that the elderly do not carry their fair share of society's workload. Unfortunately, much of the work completed by elders isn't counted. Research suggests that approximately 3 million home-care laborers would be needed if seniors stopped providing care to the sick and the disabled.[8] Such unpaid work is often hard, non-stop, grueling labor, but it's not counted except in the workbooks of heaven. Many religious institutions and volunteer-based programs would fail to operate without the help of seniors. Non-profit organizations recognize the value of and encourage senior volunteerism. Grandparenting is becoming full-time parenting for many seniors.

Surveys suggest that over a third of those over the age of 65 would prefer to work, yet they are discriminated against in competing for job positions. Many seniors forced into retirement long to be and are able to be a part of the work force. Now that we have dispelled the major myths about aging and defined more accurately the truths about it, what is successful aging?

SUCCESSFUL AGING

Some Christian seniors epitomize Ptahhotep, an Egyptian philosopher and poet who lived 2500 years before the birth of Christ. "How hard and painful are the last days of an aged man! He grows weaker every day; his eyes become dim, his ears deaf; his strength fades; his heart knows peace no longer; his mouth falls silent and he speaks no word. The power of his mind lessens and today he cannot remember what yesterday was like. All his bones hurt. Those things which not long ago were done with pleasure are painful now and taste vanishes. Old age is the worst of misfortunes that can afflict a man."[9]

One of our greatest leaders during World War II proposed a different perspective on aging:

OUTREACH
Estimate how many hours you spend each month on volunteer activities.

_____

If you were paid for these at your present hourly rate, how much money would you earn?

_____

Are you pulling your own weight in your church and community?

"Youth is not a period of time. It is a state of mind, a result of the will, a quality of the imagination, a victory of courage over timidity, of the taste of adventure over the love of comfort. A man doesn't grow old because he has lived a certain number of years. A man grows old when he deserts his ideal. The years may wrinkle his skin, but deserting his ideal wrinkles his soul. Preoccupations, fears, doubts, and despair are the enemies which slowly bow us toward earth and turn us into dust before death. You will remain young as long as you are open to what is beautiful, good, and great; receptive to the messages of other men and women, of nature and of God. If one day you should become bitter, pessimistic, and gnawed by despair, may God have mercy on your old man's soul."[10]

Rowe and Kahn's Model of Successful Aging and Positive Spirituality

In their original model based on decades of research supported by the MacArthur Foundation, Rowe and Kahn defined the key elements of successful aging as the avoidance of disease and disability, the maintenance of physical and cognitive function, and active engagement with life. Christian gerontologists have argued that positive spiritual growth represents the fourth major category of successful aging.[11] For example, spirituality has been associated with an improvement in psychological well-being, a reduction in levels of depression and distress, a reduction in disease, and an increase in life span.

Recent research helps renew the historical link between medicine and religious faith. More than 850 scientific studies have shown that faith (spirituality) enhances mental and physical health, reduces morbidity (disease), and contributes to long life.[12] The famous Johns Hopkins physician, Sir William Osler, in 1910, wrote in the first edition of the British Medical Journal, "Nothing in life is more wonderful than faith—the one great moving force which we can neither weigh in the balance nor test in the crucible."[13]

Older Christians who refuse to exercise, stop smoking, lose weight, alter their diet, or remain active socially, are on thin ice if they take seriously the teachings of Scripture. Read the verses in the margin. You may ask, *how do we change?*

We must remind ourselves to rely on God to correct aspects of our physical and emotional lifestyle. We need to believe more in God. In faith, we claim God's promises. "His divine power has given us everything we need for life and godliness through our knowledge of him who called us by his own glory and goodness. Through these he has given us his very great and precious promises, so that through them you may participate in the divine nature and escape the corruption in the world caused by evil desires" (2 Pet. 1:3-4).

As we review God's admonitions about how to age successfully, we must remind ourselves that we are saved and live by the same grace. Just as Ptahhotep's view of aging contrasts sharply with General MacAuthur's, history describes two notions of God's grace. In Martin Luther's famous debate with Erasmus on the nature of God's grace, his adversary stated that God's grace was like a parent helping a child learn to walk … the Lord helps those who help themselves. Luther countered

"Don't you know that you yourselves are God's temple and that God's Spirit lives in you? If anyone destroys God's temple, God will destroy him; for God's temple is sacred, and you are that temple."
—I Corinthians 3:16-17

"You were bought at a price. Therefore honor God with your body."
—I Corinthians 6:20

"I urge you, brothers, in view of God's mercy, to offer your bodies as living sacrifices, holy and pleasing to God—this is your spiritual act of worship."
—Romans 12:1

passionately with a word picture. " 'No, grace is a caterpillar in a ring of fire. The only deliverance is from above.' "[14]

Luther's view of the role of God's grace in our lives is that God doesn't leave us alone.

> The Lord God helps me,
> Therefore, I am not disgraced;
> Therefore, I have set My face like flint,
> And I know that I shall not be ashamed;
> He who vindicates Me is near (Isa. 50:7-8, NASB).

If we are to improve and maintain our emotional and physical health and seize His purpose for our lives no matter how old we are, we must begin with God's grace.

God's grace is realized in part when we believe that each of us has a unique, eternal mission … "the hope to which he has called you" (Eph. 1:18). What is that calling? Though I believe each of us receives a unique call from God, the mission statement for all seniors can be found in Psalm 71. Read it in the margin.

Many Christians find God's grace revealed through the lives of older friends and mentors who share their testimonies, each story laced with God's sustaining grace. Three of these great men for me are in heaven; two remain in my life. Charles faces a chronic condition called "polymyalgia rheumatica" or PMR, pain involving many muscles. This condition can produce an extremely painful swelling of the artery walls that restricts blood flow and which can cause blindness or result in a stroke. PMR has no cure. Charles also has bones that are so weakened that he could sustain a fracture just by turning over in bed. What is his mental state? "My heart is glad and my tongue rejoices; my body will also live in hope" (Acts 2:26). How is he fulfilling God's purpose for his life? Just recently, he led a 95-year-old woman to Christ.

If we are to avoid disease and minimize disability in our aging bodies, we must have an attitude of life-long learning and remain true to our spiritual mission by believing God's grace and promises. " 'I have told you these things, so that in me you may have peace. In this world you will have trouble. But take heart! I have overcome the world' " (John 16:33). The role of faith in our lives opens up a new dimension to the aging process. It enables us, enriches us, and empowers us to live beyond what we could achieve alone. "May God not find the whine in us any more, but may He find us full of spiritual pluck … ready to face anything He brings. … God never has museums."[15]

When you think of seniors, don't picture frail, dependent people. On the contrary, the hope of our nation and perhaps of the world rests on the shoulders of those who comprise the aging church. The most frail and physically dependent person may also be the most ardent prayer warrior or the most wise or courageous member of a congregation. Legions of seniors in churches nationwide can

"You have been by hope,
    O Sovereign Lord,
  my confidence since
    my youth.
From birth I have relied
    on you;
  you brought me forth from
    my mother's womb.
  I will ever praise you. …
Even when I am old and gray,
    do not forsake me, O God,
till I declare your power to
    the next generation,
  your might to all who
    are to come."
    —Psalm 71:5-6,18

lead the way to a spiritual transformation of America and even the world. Seniors can leave us a multitude of legacies, including how to:

- live sacrificially;
- appreciate traditions that teach us to value history;
- treasure the moment;
- confront our materialistic tendencies;
- value life from the womb to the grave;
- maintain a robust health and intellect for as long as possible;
- live successfully with and learn from chaos and difficulty;
- live courageously; persevere;
- express faith in love; share one's faith;
- genuinely worship;
- live on a budget;
- forgive and live in unity with other Christians;
- glorify and enjoy Christ now and forever.

[1]John W. Rowe and Robert L. Kahn, *Successful Aging* (New York: Pantheon Books, 1998), 11.
[2]Dr. Robert Butler, *Why Survive?: Being Old in America* (New York: HarperCollins Publishers, 1975) 11–15.
[3]Rowe and Kahn, *Successful Aging,* 18.
[4]Ibid., 19.
[5]Ibid., 22.
[6]Ibid., 26.
[7]Ibid., 32.
[8]Ibid., 34.
[9]Ptahhotep, as quoted in Simone de Beauvoir, *The Coming of Age,* as found in Judith Viorst, *Necessary Losses: The Loves, Illusions, Dependencies and Impossible Expectations That All of Us Have to Give Up in Order to Grow* (New York: Ballantine Books, 1986), 318.
[10]General Douglas MacArthur as quoted in James G. Daley, *Social Work Practice in the Military* (New York: Haworth Press, 1999), 255.
[11]M. Crowther, M.W. Parker, H. Koenig, W. Larimore, & A. Achenbaum, "Rowe and Kahn's Model of Successful Aging Revisited: Positive Spirituality—The Forgotten Factor," *The Gerontologist,* (in press).
[12]Ibid.
[13]Sir William Osler, "The Faith That Heals," *British Journal of Medicine,* 1910, as quoted in Walt Larimore, "Basic Spiritual Care for Patients," <*www.mercola.com/article/prayer/spiritual_care.htm*> (13 September 2002).
[14]World Harvest Mission, *Sonship* (Jenkintown, PA: World Harvest Mission, 1999).
[15]Oswald Chambers, *My Utmost for His Highest* (New York: Dodd, Mead & Company, Inc., 1935), 136.

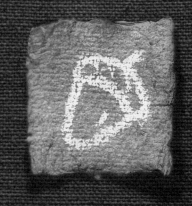

Week Nine
Lifestyle Diseases
Charles H. Elliott

Read this week's Verse to Know from Psalm 103. Ask yourself if your lifestyle blesses, or honors, God's holy name. If you are like most Americans, your lifestyle might be bringing Him dishonor while bringing you early disease. Perhaps you do lead a health conscious life but nonetheless find yourself with an unexpected disease. You probably wonder if you could have prevented or at least postponed the onset of this disease.

If your mother has high blood pressure, then will you also get high blood pressure? If your father and brother both had heart attacks before they were 50, are you next in line? All of us have questions and concerns about what impact our families' medical situations might have on our individual health. Let's look at some common diseases to see if they can be traced to lifestyle or genetics. Then let's see what you can do in either situation to lower your chances of disease.

We are told very clearly in Scripture that the Lord has a plan for each of us. We must take care of our physical bodies in order to be available to Him and His church in various areas of service.

WHAT A DIFFERENCE A CENTURY MAKES

If you were alive around the turn of the past century—1900—then you probably don't need to be reading this. You have reached the 100-year-old mark and hopefully your name and picture have appeared on television or in the local newspaper. However, for those of us who weren't around at that time, let's look at how diseases have changed. The following chart shows the difference between the five leading causes of death in the beginning and end of the 20th century.[1]

1900	1999
Pneumonia	Heart Disease
Tuberculosis	Cancer
Diarrhea and enteritis	Stroke
Heart Disease	Lung Disease
Stroke	Injury

Are you surprised to see that if you lived in the beginning of the 20th century, you would most likely die from an infection? Science has given us powerful antibiotics and vaccines that greatly decrease death and illness from bacteria and viruses. Fast forward 100 years and heart disease and cancer are the leading killers.

WHAT DO WE MEAN BY "LIFESTYLE"?

When we speak of lifestyle, we must look at many broad areas of how we live. As Christians we need to remember that everything that is within us should glorify and please our Heavenly Father. With that in mind, let's consider some lifestyle questions. Ask yourself:

- How much physical activity do I include on a regular basis?
- Do I live to eat or eat to live?
- Am I a smoker?
- Am I overweight?
- Do I have regular physical checkups?
- Do I read food labels and/or consider the fat, calorie, and sugar content of foods before I buy them?

Persons who jokingly list fried foods, gravy, potato chips, and sweets as personal basic food groups might want to consider some lifestyle changes. Let's define lifestyle as *how I live and eat every day.*

WHAT DO WE MEAN BY "GENETICS"?

We will look later at the amazing impact that the field of genetics has had on the fields of medicine and disease prevention. However, before you start getting dizzy from flashbacks to high school biology texts, we need to understand the meaning of the term *genetics.*

For purposes of our discussion, we will use a simple definition. Basically, we will consider genetics to be *the genes you inherit from your mother and father that make you who and what you are.* You have heard about DNA, RNA, genes, chromosomes, and so forth. But for our discussion, we will use the general terms *genes* or *genetics* to include all components that direct characteristics such as eye color, height, or complexion.

Around the turn of the 21st century, the Human Genome Project received a great deal of publicity. It promised to dramatically change the way we understand and treat many diseases. In the near future, your medical provider will be able to take a blood sample, run a genetic test, and determine your risk for diseases such as diabetes, asthma, heart disease, and arthritis. In addition, drug companies are feverishly working to bring us a whole new generation of medicines that are genetically based and that will be prescribed to work within your particular genetic makeup.

DISEASES—LIFESTYLE OR GENETICS?

Two leading genetic researchers, Dr. Victor McKusick, the father of genetic medicine in the 20th century and Dr. Tim Donlon of the Queens Genetics Center in

---

"Whether you eat or drink or whatever you do, do it all for the glory of God."
—1 Corinthians 10:31

UPREACH

Read Proverbs 12:1,15. Throughout the Proverbs we find encouragement to take advice while it can still do us some good. Allow God to speak to you as you continue reading this week's content. What might God be saying to you about lifestyle choices?

Hawaii, are of the opinion that all cancers and other diseases are genetically based or at least have some genetic component. In an interview in 2001, Dr. McKusick noted, "I think one can say that there is practically no disease that isn't in some measure ... genetically determined."[2] However, by our lifestyles we can often allow the "thief" into our lives to steal and destroy our health. Let's consider the lifestyle and genetic causes of four of the leading killers in the United States.

I. Cardiovascular Disease—The Leading Killer

Cardiovascular disease is the number 1 killer of both men and women. Many may find this fact surprising, especially for women, but it is true.[3]

Some key terms used to discuss cardiovascular disease are:
- Cardiovascular disease—a general term that includes coronary artery disease and other problems. Think of your arteries as a garden hose that carries blood throughout the body. Cholesterol and fats can clog up the hose much like mud and rocks do inside a hose. Or, if you prefer indoor plumbing examples, think of it as rust in a pipe. However, with either example, the arteries begin to get clogged and blood flow is reduced.
- Coronary artery disease—Your heart has three main coronary arteries which supply blood to the heart muscle. These can get clogged and shut off arteries. When that happens, it leads to death of the heart muscle. This event is called a myocardial infarction (MI) or its common name, a heart attack.
- Cholesterol—fats in the blood that can lead to "rust in the pipes."
- HDL Cholesterol—good cholesterol. It actually can act as a vacuum cleaner in the arteries and help keep them clean.
- LDL Cholesterol—bad cholesterol. It leads to blockages in the arteries.

Now let's deal with the big question, "Is cardiovascular disease caused by your lifestyle or is it genetic?" That question is best answered by taking a trip into the city of Framingham, Massachusetts. Here, over 50 years ago, researchers from the National Institutes of Health began to study the lifestyles and heart disease in about 5000 people in the city. To date, about 900 of the original members remain and many of their offspring continue to be studied. From this study an amazing amount of information has been learned about the relationship between cardiovascular disease and lifestyle. The following facts are just a few of the milestones from the Framingham study.[4] These have proven to be the basis for many current prevention and treatment recommendations.

1960—Cigarette smoking found to increase heart disease.
1961—High cholesterol and high blood pressure found to increase risk.
1967—Physical inactivity and obesity found to increase risk.
1978—Psychosocial factors (depression, alcohol abuse) found to increase risk.
1988—Higher levels of HDL cholesterol found to reduce risk of death.

Along with other studies, this research has shown a very strong relationship between lifestyle and heart disease. Now let's look at risk factors from the American Heart Association.[5]

" 'The thief comes only to steal and kill and destroy; I have come that they may have life, and have it to the full.' "
—John 10:10

INREACH
Consider the current cholesterol guidelines from the National Cholesterol Education Program of the Institutes of Health.

Total Cholesterol:
     <200 Desirable
LDL Cholesterol
     <100 Optimal
HDL Cholesterol
     >40-45 desired

If you don't know your cholesterol level, have it checked by your doctor.

OUTREACH

If you know someone who is in danger of developing a lifestyle disease, how would you approach the subject with him or her? Discuss your answer with your group.

Risk Factors You Cannot Change
- Age—The older you are, the greater your chance of a heart attack.
- Gender—Men are at greater risk and tend to have heart attacks earlier in life.
- Heredity—If your parents had heart disease, you are at greater risk.
- Race—African Americans, Native Americans, and native Hawaiians are at greater risk than Caucasians.

Risk Factors You Can Change
- Smoking—Cigarette smokers are up to four times more likely to die from a heart attack. It is the single biggest risk factor for heart disease.
- Obesity—The American Heart Association estimates that 75 percent of hypertension is caused by obesity.[6] Granted, you may have some genetic risks, but in most cases, weight is a major factor. Simply losing 10 lbs. can decrease your risk.
- Inactivity—If you are an average American, your physical activity level is low. Studies show that activity—walking, exercising, or gardening—decreases your risks.
- Cholesterol—as bad cholesterol increases, so does your risk.
- High Blood Pressure—anything above 140/90 increases your risk.
- Diabetes—diabetics have much higher risk of all cardiovascular diseases.

Genetics and Heart Disease
We wrote earlier about the Human Genome Project—what many in the scientific field consider to be one of the greatest scientific achievements of all time. In short, the scientists were able to decode our genetic code—our basic building blocks. From this, medical researchers are now discovering that diseases such as heart disease are driven by our genes as much as by our lifestyle.

We have known for many years that as many as half of heart attacks patients have normal cholesterol levels or no other risk factors. Now, genetic studies are showing that specific genes greatly increase the risk of developing heart disease.
- One research study showed that some people have genes that cause them to secrete an enzyme that protects arteries from getting clogged with disease.
- A condition known as Syndrome X appears to be genetic. It is a combination of high blood sugar, high blood pressure, high cholesterol, and obesity.
- Gene studies of mice in France showed that the fatty plaque deposits that clog arteries were eliminated when they were treated with a specific gene therapy.[7] Hopefully this research will soon lead to similar treatments for all of us!

At this time, it isn't possible to assign a percentage of lifestyle versus genetics when considering your risk for heart disease. But it appears that in a vast majority of cases, our lifestyle choices are the main factor.

Heart Disease Summary
In the opening paragraph, we asked if individuals were destined to get high blood pressure or have a heart attack because of family history. The answer appears to be a definite maybe! Clearly, the typical American lifestyle habits are contributing to

the increase of heart disease. Genetic studies continue to unfold new information that we hope one day will lead to its elimination much as we saw diseases such as smallpox eradicated. It's no longer a pipe dream. We could see this development in our lifetimes. But the central message isn't to wait on that miracle. Take care of your health on a proactive basis.

2. Cancer—The Number 2 Killer

The word *cancer* takes your breath away when directed at you or someone you love. Even though more people die from heart disease, this diagnosis often brings more fear than any other. Also, it seems to be the one set of diseases that more people ask, "What can I do to prevent it?"

Lets review some basics from the American Cancer Society to give us some perspective on this disease:

- Cancer is a group of diseases where normal cells turn abnormal and grow out of control, leading to death.
- If you look at everyone who has cancer of all types, the overall survival rate is about 60 percent. A cancer diagnosis is NOT an automatic death sentence.
- The majority of all cancers occur in those who are aged 55 or older. So, as with heart disease, the older you get, the greater your risk. However, you can be affected at any age.
- In the United States, men have a risk of about one in two of developing cancer. Women have about a one in three risk. Is this because of our lifestyles or because of genetics? Let's see what the facts indicate.

Gender and Cancer

Can you guess what cancer is the leading killer of women? If you guessed breast cancer, that is incorrect. Actually, women have reached equality with men so that now lung cancer is the leading cancer killer in women and men. I can't help but think back to the old slogan, "You've come a long way, baby." Thanks primarily to cigarettes that women smoke just like men, lung cancer is now number 1.

Breast cancer is the number 2 cancer killer of women. The third is colon and rectal cancer. We have already noted that the leading cause of cancer deaths in men is lung cancer. The second leading cause is prostate cancer. Finally, like women, colon and rectal cancer is the third leading cause of cancer deaths.

Lifestyle and Cancer

Let's look at what factors play into overall cancer risks and what we can do to decrease them.

- As with heart disease, cigarette smoking is the leading cause of cancer deaths. The American Cancer Society (ACS) estimates that in over 500,000 cancer deaths this year, smoking alone will cause about 30 percent! If you smoke, you must stop.
- The next tool the enemy uses to steal, kill, and destroy is alcohol abuse. Many cancers, especially of the gastrointestinal tract, are related to alcohol intake.

• Another ⅓ of cancers is thought to be due to poor nutrition, inactivity, obesity, and other lifestyle issues. In addition, environmental causes also may contribute to cancer deaths such as some chemicals, radiation, and toxic wastes.
• Some cancers are related to infectious exposures. These include hepatitis B virus, human papilloma virus, and human immunodeficiency virus (HIV). Many of these infections can be traced partially to sexually-transmitted diseases, a major lifestyle issue.

As an example of the power of lifestyle, the CDC studies have shown that colon cancer frequently can actually be reduced by simple physical exercise![8]

Cancer and Genetics

As with all disease, cancer has genetic components. Science is finding more genetic connections to cancers. Breast cancer patients can now be tested to see if they have the BRCA gene, which greatly increases the chances of cancer. For example, scientists have found several genes that appear to contribute to a person's susceptibility. To date, only two types of genes have been identified which seem to direct only 10 percent of colon cancer. Therefore, lifestyle appears to either cause the other cancers or at least cause a weakened gene to turn cancerous.

Cancer Summary

In the question of lifestyle versus genetics, lifestyle appears to account for the majority of cancer cases. However, that estimate is based on knowledge to date. Genetics experts believe that eventually all will be shown to have both genetic and lifestyle components.

3. Obesity

The U.S. Surgeon General declared in December 2001 that America was in the midst of an epidemic of obesity that threatens the nation's health. To give you some perspective on this issue, think about this comparison: cigarettes are thought to kill about 400,000 people a year. Obesity and the diseases it causes or worsens are now thought to cause 300,000 deaths a year! Obesity is quickly closing on cigarettes as the number 1 cause of preventable death in the United States.[9]

In 1999, over 60 percent of adults and 13 percent of children in the United Sates were considered obese—clearly a lifestyle-driven issue when you realize:
• America is the most obese, most sedentary nation in recorded history.
• High-calorie, high-fat food is available to us on a 24-hour-a-day basis.
• Serving sizes have grown to Olympian proportions. Think about the oversized plates used by most restaurants for the evening meal.
• Gluttony isn't a harmless sin. A well-known evangelist was once quoted as saying, "We are digging our own graves with our teeth." Amen!
• Our activity levels continue to drop as we become more accustomed to technology. Lack of exercise increases the frequency of several diseases.
• Just going on a diet is generally not helpful in the long run. According to the CDC, the majority of people who are attempting weight loss aren't using the correct method to achieve or maintain weight loss.[10]

"A companion of gluttons disgraces his father."
—Proverbs 28:7

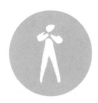

INREACH

Controlling the portion sizes you eat is a great way to control calorie intake. Consistently read labels and eat the recommended serving sizes.

Genetics and Obesity

Several genetic factors are being investigated. About seven genetic mutations have been linked to severe obesity. In terms of medical conditions, a few could contribute to obesity such as hypothyroidism, Cushings Disease, and polycystic ovarian syndrome. However, authorities consider the most common cause of obesity in the United States to be individual lifestyle choices, not genetic predetermination.

4. Diabetes

We are experiencing an explosion in the number of diabetics according to the American Diabetes Association. Let's review some basic information about diabetes to have a better understanding of the disease.

Glucose (sugar) comes from the foods we eat. Glucose is the body's main fuel source. Cells make up all parts of our bodies, and they need the energy that glucose provides. Insulin produced by the pancreas assists glucose into the cells so that it can be used. It must be present and working properly to move glucose from the bloodstream and into most cells.

Diabetics either don't make enough insulin or cannot use their insulin properly. The glucose may get too high (hyperglycemia) or too low (hypoglycemia). High levels of glucose can damage blood vessels, nerve endings, and organs, causing long-term complications.

Diabetes has no cure; it is a lifelong health problem. Borderline diabetes is a myth. If blood glucose is ever measured over 200, that person has diabetes. Proper treatment that is lifelong and consistent can help control high blood glucose.

Types of diabetes:

Type 1 diabetes used to be called *Insulin Dependent Diabetes,* since anyone with this disease had to take insulin injections to supply what the body didn't produce or have in enough supply. One out of ten diabetics has type 1, and a genetic trait must be present to get it. People with type 1 usually are thin or normal weight and are under age 30 when diagnosed. The pancreas doesn't make insulin, and daily injections must be taken so that food can be used by the cells and not stored as fat which isn't a good fuel source for energy. Type 1 diabetes can be controlled by taking daily insulin, following a meal and exercise plan, and monitoring blood glucose routinely.

With type 2 diabetes, the insulin no longer works as well to get the glucose into the body's cells, so blood glucose gets high. Some of the glucose continues to move into the body's cells, but not enough. Type 2 diabetics frequently are overweight, have a family history of diabetes, are over age 45, have a history of diabetes during pregnancy, or have high blood pressure. Type 2 diabetes begins and progresses slowly; many who have the disease don't know it. Type 2 diabetes is best controlled by following a meal and exercise plan and monitoring blood glucose routinely. Medication such as pills or insulin injections may be required to keep the diabetes under control.[12]

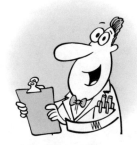

Professor Phitt asks:

Can you name the primary symptoms of diabetes?

• Frequent urination
• Excessive thirst
• Extreme hunger
• Unusual weight loss
• Increased fatigue
• Irritability
• Blurry vision

If you have one or more of these symptoms, see your doctor right away.[11]

OUTREACH

Share what you have
learned in this chapter with
members of your family.
Remember to set a good
example for your family.

Diabetes is the leading cause of blindness and kidney failure in the United States.[13] Also, it increases the risk for heart attack and stroke. It can lead to poor circulation which, if untreated, can lead to loss of toes, feet, fingers, and so forth.

Lifestyle vs. Genetics in Diabetes

As with the previous diseases, research is showing many genetically-driven components, especially to type 1 diabetes. However, both types are clearly being driven by our lifestyles of low activity and high-calorie foods, a dangerous combination Some known genetic factors are at play, but even so, control of blood sugar, lifestyle adjustments, and sometimes medication are essential.

Summary of Lifestyle vs. Genetics in Disease

We have reviewed heart disease, cancer, obesity, and diabetes and the areas that are impacted by lifestyle vs. genetics. Genetic experts argue that eventually all diseases will be shown to have a genetic component, but our lifestyles of inactivity, obesity, high-calorie foods, and other factors appear to be driving a great majority of preventable diseases. We must present our bodies as "living sacrifices" (Rom. 12:1) to the Lord and start taking care of our physical bodies. Remember, it is much more difficult to regain health when you lose it than to keep it while you are healthy.

In closing, keep in mind God's promise for your future and don't allow your personal health choices to impact this negatively.

---

[1]Adapted from National Center for Health Statistics, "The 10 Leading Causes of Death," <*www.ncsl.org/ programs/health/marks/sld003.htm*> (17 September 2002), and Donna L. Hoyert et at., "Deaths: Final Data for 1999," *National Vital Statistics Reports,* 49:8 (21 September 2001).

[2]Victor McKusick, "Victor McKusick: Genetic Medicine in the 21st Century—What's Ahead?" <*www.dna.com/eventTranscripts/eventTranscript_jsp?link=200105041100.htm*> (17 January 2002).

[3]American Heart Association, "2002 Heart and Stroke Statistical Update" (Dallas, TX: American Heart Association, 2001), 6, as cited in <*www.americanheart.org/presenter/jhtml?identifier=1928*> (3 August 2002).

[4]Framingham Heart Study, "Research Milestones," <*www.nhlbi.nih.gov/about/framingham/timeline.htm*> (24 February 2002).

[5]American Heart Association, "Risk Factors for Coronary Heart Disease," <*http://216.185.112.5/presenter. jhtml?identifier=2357*> (12 September 2002).

[6]American Heart Association, "Obesity: Impact on Cardiovascular Disease," <*http://216.185.112.5/presenter.jhtml?identifier=1818*> (12 September 2002).

[7]Caroline Desurmont, et al., "Complete Atherosclerosis Regression After Human ApoE Gene Transfer in ApoE–Deficient/Nude Mice," Arteriosclerosis, Thrombosis, and Vascular Biology: Journal of the American Heart Association 20 (2000): 435.

[8]Center for Disease Control, "How Physical Activity Impacts Health," <*www.cdc.gov/nccdphp/sgr/mm.htm*> (13 September 2002).

[9]The American Cancer Society, *Cancer Facts and Figures,* 2001, 23,29.

[10]Center for Disease Control, "Overweight and Obesity: Frequently Asked Questions," <*www.cdc.gov/ nccdphp/dnpa/obesity/faq.htm*> (13 September 2002).

[11]American Diabetes Association, "Symptoms," <*www.diabetes.org/main/info/diagnosed/symptoms/default.jsp*> (12 September 2002).

[12]Diabetes Healthways[SM] *Patient Education Manual,* (Nashville: American Healthways, Inc., 2001), 9-13.

[13]Center for Disease Control, "National Diabetes Fact Sheet," <*www.cdc.gov/diabetes/pubs/estimates.htm#complications*> (13 September 2002).

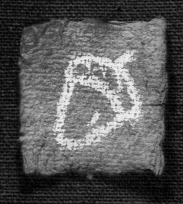

Week 10
CAM Therapies
Charles H. Elliott

Perhaps you are one of the millions of people who have used a complementary or alternative medicine or therapy within the past year. Or, maybe you hear about acupuncture, yoga, massage therapy, and other treatment options and want to know if these are safe and effective. You may question if a Christian should participate in these and similar avenues of care. Join us as we look at these and other types of CAM (Complementary and Alternative Medicine) prevention and care.

DEFINITIONS OF COMMON TERMS

Let's learn the language of the field and understand what the more common terms mean. Here are some of the basics of CAM.

- Alternative Medicine—care or prevention of a disease or condition that is done instead of traditional medical care (TMC). An example would be seeing a chiropractor instead of your family doctor for back pain.
- Complementary Medicine—care or prevention of a disease or condition that is done along with TMC. An example would be using acupuncture to assist with the nausea from chemotherapy.
- Traditional Medical Care—care or prevention of a disease that is based upon standard mainstream medical principles. An example would be muscle relaxants and pain medication prescribed by your family doctor for back pain.
- Medical Studies—research that has been printed in a medical journal. Make sure the care you receive has been adequately studied and is both safe and effective. As a general rule, at least one study somewhere will support a theory or new idea about medical care. Beware headlines that say, "Study Shows Cure for Disease X." Results from a very poor study would mean little.
- Double-Blind Study—the highest level of medical study that is the gold standard to see whether something works. Two groups of people were studied. One received a type of care; the other didn't receive the same care. No one, including the doctors, knew which group they were in, hence the term *blind*. An example is a study in which women are given pill A or pill B each day. These women and their doctors don't know what they have been given until the study is done and results compared.

- Placebo Effect–a medical effect a person receives from a suggestion of care. For example, you could give someone with a headache a placebo pill that has nothing in it. However, the headache goes away because the patient believes in the power of the empty pill. The pain relief results from the placebo effect.
- Bias–a feeling of how something should be without actually studying the facts. For example, I might have a bias toward traditional therapies because they have been proven to be effective. But I don't actually investigate my positions; I act on biased feelings because I feel comfortable with them.

 Can you draw a line to match these terms with their definitions?

• CAM	published in a medical journal
• TMC	a feeling rather than a medical proof
• medical studies	medical effect from the suggestion of care
• double blind study	complementary and alternative medicine
• placebo effect	two trial groups
• bias	traditional medicine

OUTREACH
Have you been part of a medical study? If so, be prepared to share your experience with your group.

Now you know the basic language of CAM. Since I have spent more than 20 years in the field of traditional medical care (TMC), you might argue that I am biased toward this field. However, I have made every effort to present a balanced view of the following information. Since an increasing number of patients are using CAM, I have seen both good and bad results. In all fairness, I have also seen good and bad results from TMC.

Let's approach this topic by looking through the eyes of a Christian who wants good information. Keep in mind that neither the writer nor *Fit 4: The LifeWay Christian Wellness Plan* endorses any of the following therapies.

The National Center for Complementary and Alternative Medicine
As the number of questions grows about effectiveness and safety of CAM, the federal government is leading the way in producing major studies. In 1998, under the renowned National Institutes of Health (NIH), the National Center for Complementary and Alternative Medicine was established with a current budget of about $100 million. Its purpose is to develop and support unbiased medical research related to CAM for the benefit of the public. Its overriding mission is to provide reliable information about the safety and effectiveness of CAM practices. Much of the information in this review is a result of NCCAM studies to date.

CAM's Growing Popularity in the United States
Current studies estimate that about 50 percent of American adults use some sort of CAM, and the number is growing rapidly. As it continues to grow in popularity, investigators are trying to determine how and why people use CAM. According to a major study in 1998, people who use CAM tend to have a holistic philosophy of health.[1] The health of body, mind and spirit are related, and whoever takes care of health should treat the whole person.

You may have noted the similarity between this viewpoint and the biblically-based philosophy of *Fit 4,* which supports a holistic look at health. Our *Fit 4* theme verses remind us to love God with our hearts, souls, minds, and strength (Mark 12:30).

In week 3, you were introduced to natural remedies and herbal medicine, so we won't review these elements of CAM. This week we will examine some of the more popular forms of CAM: chiropractic, acupuncture, massage, yoga, and chelation therapy. Some insurance companies are becoming more accepting of CAM care, providing coverage for some alternative treatments. Doors are opening.

CHIROPRACTIC

One of the more popular CAM therapies in use, chiropractic has grown to the point that chiropractors report 20 million patient visits a year in the United States. While acceptance by the public has grown, relations with traditional medical providers remain a problem in many areas. TMC providers argue that no major valid studies document chiropractic care as effective for anything other than short-term low-back pain. "But as a treatment act, it has gained wide acceptance."[2] Patients continue to believe in the care they receive. They tend to rate their satisfaction with chiropractic care higher than their TMC providers.

Numerous studies have shown chiropractic care to be effective and safe for a variety of conditions. "In 1994, the Agency for Health Care Policy and Research (AHCPR), a branch of the U.S. Department of Health and Human Services, recommended spinal manipulation as an initial form of therapy for low back sufferers, finding it both 'safe and effective.' "[3] "The statement by AHCPR was based on its scientific review of all the accumulated evidence on spinal manipulation. Spinal manipulation is the primary form of treatment performed by doctors of chiropractic. In fact, doctors of chiropractic perform 94 percent of all spinal manipulative therapy in the United States."[4]

A study published in the 1995 British Medical Journal study concluded, " 'The beneficial effect of chiropractic on pain was particularly clear.' "[5] More recently, a study released in 2001 by the Center for Clinical Health Policy Research at Duke University concluded that "spinal manipulation resulted in almost immediate improvement for cervicogenic headaches, or those that originate in the neck, and had significantly fewer side effects and longer-lasting relief of tension-type headache than a commonly prescribed medication."[6]

A typical chiropractic visit requires about 20 minutes for spinal manipulation and other related treatments. Usually, the patient is rescheduled for visits during the next several weeks for the chiropractor to evaluate the effectiveness of the therapy. Some chiropractors stay within the standard Palmer spinal treatment protocols while others may branch out into more general treatments. Some claim to help various problems such as menstrual irregularity, headaches, and low immune systems, although to date I'm not aware of any studies that have shown these treatments to be effective.

INREACH

Holistic health is whole-person health. From your own experience, give an example of the connection between your emotions, mind, spirit, and body.

A federal government supported study published in 1998 studied 321 adult low-back patients who were assigned to one of three treatments: 1) Chiropractic, 2) Physical Therapy (McKenzie Method), and 3) education (given a booklet to read about back pain and released). The results showed that people who were just given a booklet did as well physically as the other two. Their progress was followed for a year afterward. However, those who went to both the chiropractors and physical therapists did rate their satisfaction higher.[7] This study raises the possibility that the placebo effect may have been a factor in perceived benefits.

Despite results of favorable studies, opponents continue to question the legitimacy of chiropractic care, noting the risks of cervical (neck) manipulation. Proponents counter that TMC also faces risks of adverse drug reactions which each year result in patient deaths or serious side effects.

ACUPUNCTURE

Acupuncture is one of the oldest medical procedures in the world, originating in China over 2000 years ago. It became more widely known in America in 1972 when a reporter accompanying President Nixon to China had to have an emergency appendectomy. Acupuncture was used to help him with pain, so the story spread via the press.

Acupuncture, one of the more accepted CAM treatments, has shown effectiveness in medical studies—especially pain syndromes and nausea related to chemotherapy or surgical anesthesia. In most of these cases, it's used to complement standard care. Studies have shown that in many cases less pain medication is needed.

When acupuncture began, study of the human body by dissection was forbidden, so Chinese physicians determined that energy flow was central to health. They believed the body has energy pathways called meridians that conduct energy, or *qi,* (pronounced *chee),* According to these practitioners, opposing forces in the body influence *qi*. The acupuncture needles are inserted into the skin at any of more than 2000 acupuncture points to keep the normal flow of *qi* unblocked. Most Western doctors use acupuncture because of proven benefits and not because of the philosophy from which it came.

Some acupuncturists offer herbal treatment as part of a session. If you are given this option, use extreme caution and discuss it with your TMC physician before using the herbs internally. They could interact with medications you are taking or cause side effects. In addition, make sure to ask that your acupuncturist use only clean, disposable needles.

Many who offer TMC are beginning to add acupuncture as part of patient care. However, a gap remains between the two fields of TMC and CAM, as much of the effect of acupuncture can't be explained in the traditional Western medical way of thinking. At this point, the NCCAM is funding several clinical studies to determine if acupuncture is actually safe and effective. However, its use often depends on whether insurance will reimburse for it.

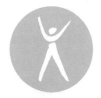

UPREACH
Read Philippians 1:9-11. Use discernment, or good judgment, when considering a CAM. Prayerfully allow God to direct your choices.

MASSAGE

This field includes a broad range of practitioners, including therapeutic massage, reflexology, lymphatic massage, craniosacral therapy, and many others. I am using the term *massage* in a generic sense to mean manipulation of soft tissues in the body. The skin is the body's largest organ, and touch is the first sense to develop in humans. Touch therapy has been shown to be beneficial for premature infants and autistic children, among others.[8]

Basically, this field involves a practitioner massaging an area of the body to release various problems that arise. These blockages include muscle trigger points, poor circulation, lymph flow problems, or connective tissue or other muscle tension areas. According to practitioners, massage:

- relieves stress;
- lifts depression;
- increases circulation in the body;
- reduces muscle fatigue;
- boosts the immune system;
- clears the respiratory area;
- reduces/removes migraines and other headaches;
- creates a better sleep pattern.

The University of Miami School of Medicine's Touch Research Institute (TRI) brings together researchers from several major universities to study the sense of touch and how it might be used to promote health and treat disease. So far, TRI has uncovered surprising evidence that touch can aid the healing process.[9]

Craniosacral therapy is relatively new. Developed in 1970 by John Upledger, it involves freeing up restrictions of cerebrospinal fluid along the spine.[10] Reflexology commonly focuses on the reflex points of the feet, hands, and ears. It has been used in China as a healing therapy for many thousands of years. By applying firm pressure with the thumb to specific nerve endings in the foot, an impulse is conveyed causing a reflex response. This stimulates organs such as pituitary glands, lungs, bladder, kidneys, stomach, and spleen to return to optimal functioning. The therapist deeply massages the appropriate site on the foot to stimulate and restore the free flow of energy in ten zonal pathways.

In general, massage therapies are safe and effective for relaxation. Studies are ongoing for experiments and research into the healing effects of therapeutic touch. I'm not aware of studies that show massage has curative effects on actual underlying disease. Therefore, if pain continues, see a TMC practitioner to assure that no serious illness is the source of pain.

YOGA

The word *yoga* is derived from a Sanskrit word meaning *union*. Considered to be centuries old, yoga is an integral part of the Hindu religion. Many types exist, and each attempts to make connection between body, mind, and spirit. As part of the Hindu religion, it seeks union with the divine. Although some yoga practitioners

Defining Massage

Deep tissue—releases the chronic patterns of tension in the body through slow strokes and deep finger pressure on the contracted areas.

Sports Massage—massage therapy focusing on muscle systems relevant to a particular sport.

Swedish Massage—a system of long strokes, kneading and friction techniques on the more superficial layers of the muscles, combined with active and passive movements of the joints.

Trigger Point Therapy—applies concentrated finger pressure to "trigger points" (painful irritated areas in the muscles) to break cycles of spasm and pain.

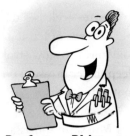

Professor Phitt says:

To find out more about the importance of flexibility and balance read or review Week 6 in the *Fit 4 Fitness* member workbook, pages 51-56. Try the flexibility exercises on page 57.

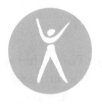

UPREACH

How would you counter the spiritual claims of yoga? (Read John 14:6.)

concentrate on the exercises spiritual aspects, others treat it as a means to gain flexibility and relaxation. Yoga incorporates three major techniques:

- Breathing lessons called *pranayma*, thought to increase blood circulation and deep breathing as well as to decrease stress.
- Physical postures called *asanas* designed to regulate the flow of energy, called *prana*, the Hindu word for life energy. You may have seen some of the numerous positions for these exercises.
- Meditation—Christians must raise a red flag at this point. Although a person might begin yoga at a basic level simply for flexibility and stress reduction, spiritual "enlightenment" will eventually be incorporated by most yoga teachers. In the book *Alternative Medicine: The Christian Handbook*, the authors explain in detail what the meditation and spirituality of yoga seeks to attain. Basically, the pinnacle of spiritual enlightenment of yoga is called "kundalini arousal." "In Hindu mythology, Kundalini is the serpent goddess who rests at the base of the spine." When aroused, the serpent travels up the spine, activating the *prana* life energy. This "releases psychic abilities, including healing powers." When Kundalini reaches the head, the person is open to enlightenment from occult sources and spirit guides.[11] Clearly, this belief is in direct conflict with Christian Scripture. (See Leviticus 19:26,31 and 2 Chronicles 33:6.)

Several studies have shown that yoga improves physical fitness and flexibility when used consistently. Also, some studies suggest help from yoga for chronic pain relief and asthma. However, I'm not aware of studies that show it decreases or stops disease. It's considered to be generally good for the body in most cases. In many communities it's almost trendy to attend yoga classes.

As previously noted, Christians need to avoid the spiritual side of yoga. However, I have had personal communications with Christians who use the breathing and physical portions while listening to Christian music or as a time of personal prayer to the name above all names, the name of Jesus. "For from him and through him and to him are all things. To him be the glory forever! Amen" (Rom. 11:36). Keep that in mind while you do your stretches.

CHELATION THERAPY

In week 9 on Lifestyle Diseases, I attempted to explain cardiovascular disease. Basically, it's like rust in a pipe. The more you have clogging your arteries, the greater your risk of heart disease. The clogging in the arteries is made up of fat and calcium. With that in mind, understand that chelation therapy tries to rid the artery of the blockages, or to clean the calcium out of the pipe. This type of CAM can have serious side effects. One of the most serious effects is that a person with significant heart disease who uses this therapy instead of traditional medical care is putting his or her life at risk.

The history of chelation is actually based in traditional medical care, so many people assume it is safe. Decades ago, it was determined that if a person had lead poisoning, the doctor could put a chemical called EDTA into the bloodstream. The EDTA acted like a claw (*chele* is Greek for *claw)* and took the lead out of the bloodstream. Also around that time, the United States Navy was using EDTA to clean calcium out of real pipes that were in boilers. The clogging in the boilers was due to calcium, and EDTA helped rid it from the pipes in engines and boilers.[12]

Then, a doctor concluded that if EDTA worked to remove lead from the bloodstream, and it removed calcium from engine and boiler pipes, why not use EDTA in humans to remove calcium from the arteries (human pipes)? In the late 1950s, he began using chelation to fight the blockages in the arteries.[13]

Today, in spite of opposition from the Food and Drug Administration, the American College of Cardiology, the American Heart Association, the American College of Physicians, and numerous other national medical groups, chelation therapy continues. Again, I'm not aware of valid medical studies that show any positive effect from chelation therapy on cardiovascular disease. In fact, a recent study entitled "Chelation Therapy for Ischemic Heart Disease" was published in the Journal of the American Medical Association.[14] The authors followed 84 patients for 27 weeks. The well-designed, double blind study showed no beneficial effect from chelation therapy.

A course of chelation therapy resembles that of a kidney dialysis patient. The patient is given an IV for three to four hours at a time for dozens of times over a one- to two-month period. Insurance doesn't cover this therapy, so one could spend thousands of dollars on a procedure that virtually all medical authorities consider useless if not dangerous.

If you are considering chelation therapy, have an in-depth discussion with your TMC physician, preferably a cardiologist. If, after that, you decide to go ahead with this therapy, make sure your chelation doctor sends regular reports to your TMC physician so he or she is kept well aware of your status.

CAM SUMMARY

We have now reviewed several of the more commonly used CAM therapies, not including the nutritional and herbal supplements, which were covered in week 3. As Christians, we want to take care of our health as good stewards of the life God has given us. On the one hand, we want to be wary of unproven therapies.

I watched my mother die a long painful death related to Alzheimer's, and my father died from cardiovascular disease. As a medical practitioner, I see regularly what disease can do to a person. If traditional medical care doesn't work as we want, we can easily become victims of those who present a new, special treatment as the answer. I urge caution. Read 2 Timothy 4:3-4 in the margin.

On the other hand, I don't intend to indict all CAM practices or practitioners. I will strongly support the NCCAM studies which will be released over the next few years. I trust many of these will show us that some CAM therapies are as safe and as effective as TMC. However, until we know the truth in these matters, I urge you to watch carefully for what I call "Charlie's Top Five CAM Red Flags."

"The time will come when men will not put up with sound doctrine. Instead, to suit their own desires, they will gather around them a great number of teachers to say what their itching ears want to hear. They will turn their ears away from the truth and turn aside to myths."
—2 Timothy 4:3-4

Charlie's Top Five CAM Red Flags

Red Flag 1—You are involved in CAM without telling your traditional medical care physician. Always keep your TMC doctor aware of what you are doing.

Red Flag 2—You take herbal supplements or nutritional aids without telling your TMC physician. These are generally unregulated, uncontrolled substances that can have serious side effects and interfere with prescription medications. As a rule, be skeptical about claims of energy boosts and other desired effects.

Red Flag 3—Your CAM provider tells you he or she needs to see you for multiple visits over several months. This schedule may be driven by a need for extended income for the provider! Although some TMC therapies involve a course of regularly scheduled treatments, these are based on valid medical studies.

Red Flag 4—Don't be swayed simply because your CAM provider claims to be a Christian. Our natural response is to trust a fellow believer. Your CAM provider must not take advantage of you or your situation with unproven therapies.

Red Flag 5—You must feel free to ask questions and to get assurances from both TMC and CAM providers that they are guarding your personal safety. The first rule of medicine is "First, do no harm."

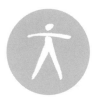

OUTREACH

Write an encouraging note to your *Fit 4* facilitator thanking him or her for leading your group session each week.

[1] John A. Astin, "Why Patients Use Alternative Medicine; Results of a National Study," *Journal of the American Medical Association,* 279 (1998):1548–53.

[2] N. M. Hadler, "Complementary and Alternative Therapies for Rheumatic Diseases II," *Rheumatic Disease Clinics of North America,* 26 (2000): 97–102.

[3] S. Bigos, et al. "Acute Low Back Problems in Adults." *Clinical practice guidelines no. 14 AHCPR Publication No. 95-0642.* (Rockville, MD: Agency for Health Care Policy and Research, Public Health Service, U.S. Department of Health and Human Services, Dec. 1994), as quoted in Daryl D. Wills, letter to Pat Mitchell, 7 June 2002, as cited on <*www.amerchiro.org/hot_topics/060702.shtml*> (3 September 2002).

[4] Shekelle, et al. "The Appropriateness of Spinal Manipulation for Low Back Pain: Project Overview and Literature Review," (RAND, R-4025/1-CCR, 1991), n. pag., as quoted in Daryl D. Wills, letter to Pat Mitchell, 7 June 2002, as cited on <*www.amerchiro.org/hot_topics/060702.shtml*> (3 September 2002).

[5] T. Meade, et at., "Randomized Comparison of Chiropractic and Hospital Outpatient Management of Low Back Pain: Results From an Extended Followup," (*British Medical Journal,* 1995), 311:349–351, as quoted in Daryl D. Wills, letter to Pat Mitchell, 7 June 2002, as cited on <*www.amerchiro.org/hot_topics/060702.shtml*> (3 September 2002).

[6] DC McCrory, et al., "Evidence Report: Behavioral and Physical Treatments for Tension-Type and Cervicogenic Headache," (Des Moines, IA: Foundation for Chiropractic Education and Research, 2001), as quoted in Daryl D. Wills, letter to Pat Mitchell, 7 June 2002, <*www.amerchiro.org/hot_topics/060702.shtml*> (3 September 2002).

[7] Daniel Cherkin et al., "Comparisons of Physical Therapy, Chiropractic Manipulation, and Provision of an Educational Booklet for the Treatment of Patients with Low Back Pain," *New England Journal of Medicine* 339 (1998), 1021–29.

[8] Tom McNichol, "The Power of Touch," *USA Weekend,* 6-8 February 1996, 22.

[9] Ibid.

[10] John Greenwald, "[Craniosacral Therapy] A New Kind of Pulse," *Time,* 16 April 2001, 68–69.

[11] Adapted from Donal O'Mathuna and Walt Larimore, *Alternative Medicine: The Christian Handbook,* (Grand Rapids, MI: Zondervan Publishing House, 2001), 285–87.

[12] Ibid., 161–63.

[13] Ibid.

[14] Merril L. Knudtson et al., "Chelation Therapy for Ischemic Heart Disease: A Randomized Controlled Trial," *Journal of American Medical Association,* 287 (2002): 481–86.

TOTAL WELLNESS LIFESTYLE ASSESSMENT

Total wellness is a combination of emotional/relational, spiritual, mental, and physical health. The following assessment is a broad stroke analysis of your lifestyle progress toward total wellness. It can also serve as a guideline for your wellness journey. This tool will evaluate your progress, but it is not meant for you to judge or belittle yourself. We all have areas where we are strong and others that need improvement. Only Jesus would get a perfect score (1 Peter 1:19)!

Instructions:

STEP I
Read the statements on each of the wellness assessments on pages 90-93. Honestly evaluate each statement without judging yourself or rationalizing your response.

- DO check the box beside each statement that is true for you virtually all the time.

- DO check the box if the statement does not apply to you. (You get credit if the statement does not apply or will never happen for you. Example: If you are an only child, put a check mark beside the statement "I get along well with my sibling(s)" because there is nothing you can do to alter this situation to make the statement true or not for you.)

- DO NOT check the box if the statement is untrue, partially true, inconsistent in your lifestyle, or you do not know the answer.

Disclaimer:

This is your personal assessment. You will not be asked to share specific answers with anyone unless you choose to do so. This assessment is for adults only and should not be used to evaluate children and teens who have different sleep, nutrition, and physical needs; are largely dependent emotionally and relationally on others in a way that is appropriate for the age group; and who may not have reached the age/ability to understand spiritual concepts related to salvation and the Christian life.

ASSESSING YOUR EMOTIONAL/RELATIONAL WELLNESS

❑ I have told my parents that I love them within the last three months.

❑ I get along well with my sibling(s).

❑ I get along well with my coworkers/clients.

❑ I get along well with my manager/staff.

❑ I get along well with my neighbors.

❑ I have a circle of friends/family that love and appreciate me for who I am, more than just what I do for them.

❑ There is no one who I would dread or feel uncomfortable coming across (in the street, at an airport or social event) at any time.

❑ I put people first and results second.

❑ I have mended or attempted to mend relationships with anyone whom I have offended, injured, or seriously disturbed, even if it wasn't fully my fault.

❑ I express my anger in non-violent ways.

❑ I receive enough love from people around me.

❑ I have a best friend or soul mate relationship with another person.

❑ I handle/manage my negative emotions in nondestructive ways.

❑ I am a person of his/her word; people can count on me.

❑ I quickly clear miscommunications and misunderstandings when they occur.

❑ I am genuinely happy for those who have achieved accomplishments, rewards and goals in their lives.

❑ I am personally responsible for my level of happiness and satisfaction in life.

❑ People feel comfortable in my home.

❑ I am in an accountability relationship with another person that I can trust.

❑ I identify, understand, and communicate my emotions when they occur.

❑ I can identify most emotions in other people.

❑ I do not dwell on emotional pain from my past.

❑ I have established and enforce healthy boundaries in all of my relationships.

❑ I do not live with persistent shame for past poor choices.

❑ I understand my personality type and the accompanying strengths and weaknesses.

_____ Number of checked items

ASSESSING YOUR SPIRITUAL WELLNESS

❑ I know, without a doubt, that I have accepted Christ as my Savior.

❑ I am an active member in a local, biblically-sound church.

❑ I have a daily Bible study and prayer time.

❑ I am growing spiritually in my walk with Christ.

❑ I seek to understand what I believe and why I believe it.

❑ I openly share my faith with others.

❑ I use biblical truths to make decisions at work.

❑ I have a strong moral foundation based on the Bible.

❑ I tithe at least 10 percent of my monthly income.

❑ I am involved in a small group Bible study or Sunday School class.

❑ I do not gossip or talk about others.

❑ I tell the truth, no matter what.

❑ I do not judge or criticize others.

❑ I have forgiven those people who have hurt/damaged me, deliberate or not.

❑ I seek God's guidance when making decisions in my personal life.

❑ I pray many times during the day.

❑ I have a spiritual mentor who helps me grow in my faith.

❑ I memorize Scripture verses or passages.

❑ I am joyful in spite of my circumstances.

❑ I seek godly counsel from other believers.

❑ I know I am valuable to God.

❑ I know God has a plan and purpose for my life even if it is not clear now.

❑ I am convicted by my sin and immediately confess it and receive forgiveness.

❑ I know and understand my spiritual gifts and minister to others from this giftedness.

❑ I have a regularly scheduled time of solitude and spiritual reflection.

_____ Number of checked items

ASSESSING YOUR PHYSICAL WELLNESS

❑ I know my body is the temple of the Holy Spirit and make healthful choices to honor God.

❑ I exercise at least three times per week.

❑ I limit caffeine intake (chocolate, coffee, colas, tea) to less than three times per week.

❑ I limit high sugar food choices to less than three times per week.

❑ I do not drink alcohol in any form.

❑ My cholesterol count is within a healthful range.

❑ My blood pressure is within a healthful range.

❑ I have had a complete physical exam in the past three years.

❑ I do not smoke/use tobacco products.

❑ My weight is within a healthful range.

❑ My nails and hair are clean and healthy.

❑ I do not use illegal drugs or misuse prescribed medications.

❑ I have had a complete eye exam within the past two years.

❑ I am aware of the physical challenges or conditions I have and am now fully taking care of them.

❑ I eat fruit everyday.

❑ I eat colorful vegetables everyday.

❑ I eat fried foods no more than once a week.

❑ I readily try new and different food in my eating plan.

❑ I hear well.

❑ I have had a dental checkup within the last year.

❑ My teeth are healthy. I brush and floss daily.

❑ I get 6-8 hours of sleep every night.

❑ I do resistance/strength training at least two times a week.

❑ My joints and muscles are flexible; I can move freely without limitations.

❑ I do not live with chronic pain.

_____ Number of checked items

ASSESSING YOUR MENTAL WELLNESS

❏ I am willing to learn new things.

❏ I have written goals, and I focus on accomplishing them.

❏ I have something to look forward to virtually every day.

❏ I consistently take evenings, weekends and holidays off from work and take at least two weeks of vacation each year.

❏ I know how much I must have to be minimally financially secure.

❏ I have no habits which I find to be unacceptable.

❏ I rarely watch television. (Less than six hours per week.)

❏ I do not rush or use adrenaline to get a job done.

❏ My personal files, papers, and receipts are neatly filed away.

❏ My home is free of clutter. I have nothing around the house or in storage that I do not need or love.

❏ I surround myself with music which makes my life more enjoyable.

❏ I am consistently early or easily on time.

❏ My work environment is productive and inspiring (ample tools and resources; no excessive pressure; organized and neat).

❏ My home is organized and well kept.

❏ I can mentally unwind in my home.

❏ I currently live well within my financial means.

❏ I have a system in place to accomplish tasks each day.

❏ I have no loose ends at work.

❏ I mentally prepare for changes in life and adapt to them successfully.

❏ I identify painful memories and learn from them without dwelling on them.

❏ I have a healthy view of myself without comparing myself to others.

❏ I keep my thoughts focused on the right things.

❏ I have a positive outlook on life.

❏ I seek solutions to problems and challenges rather than dwelling on the problem and being victimized by it.

❏ I seek to have the mind of Christ.

_____ Number of checked items

TOTAL WELLNESS ASSESSMENT EVALUATION

STEP 2: Total each section by counting the number of checked statements. Add all the totals for each section for a total wellness score. (Maximum score 100 pts.)

_____ Total true statements for all four sections

STEP 3: Shade in the progress chart below. Start from the bottom and shade one space for each point you scored in each category. You now have a current picture of how you are doing in each of the four areas. You may choose to set goals based on the areas that need improvement.

Date of first assessment: _____

Emotional Wellness	Physical Wellness	Mental Wellness	Spiritual Wellness

TOTAL WELLNESS PROGRESS CHART

STEP 4: Reevaluate your progress based on your goals in three months, six months and one year by taking the assessment over again. Record your progress on the lines provided on the evaluation page.

	Date	Points (+/-)	Total Score
Current	_____	_____	_____
3 months	_____	_____	_____
6 months	_____	_____	_____
1 year	_____	_____	_____

Read the Bible Through

JANUARY
1 Gen. 1—3; Matt. 1
2 Gen. 4—6; Matt. 2:1-12
3 Gen. 7—8; Matt. 2:13-23
4 Gen. 9—11; Matt. 3
5 Gen. 12—14; Matt. 4:1-11
6 Gen. 15—17; Matt. 4:12-25
7 Gen. 18—19; Matt. 5:1-16
8 Gen. 20—22; Matt. 5:17-48
9 Gen. 23—24; Matt. 6:1-18
10 Gen. 25—27; Matt. 6:19-34
11 Gen. 28—29 Matt. 7:1-14
12 Gen. 30—31; Matt. 7:15-29
13 Gen. 32—33; Matt. 8:1-17
14 Gen. 34—36; Matt. 8:18-34
15 Gen. 37—38; Matt. 9:1-26
16 Gen. 39—40; Matt. 9:27-38
17 Gen. 41—42; Matt. 10
18 Gen. 43—45; Matt. 11:1-19
19 Gen. 46—47; Matt. 11:20-30
20 Gen. 48—50; Matt. 12:1-21
21 Ex. 1—2; Matt. 12:22-50
22 Ex. 3—4; Matt. 13:1-23
23 Ex. 5—7; Matt. 13:24-58
24 Ex. 8—9; Matt. 14:1-21
25 Ex. 10—11; Matt. 14:22-36
26 Ex. 12—13; Matt. 15:1-20
27 Ex. 14—15; Matt. 15:21-39
28 Ex. 16—18; Matt. 16:1-12
29 Ex. 19—21; Matt. 16:13-28
30 Ex. 22—23; Matt. 17:1-13
31 Ex. 24—26; Matt. 17:14-27

FEBRUARY
1 Ex. 27—28; Matt. 18:1-20
2 Ex. 29—30; Matt. 18:21-35
3 Ex. 31—32; Matt. 19:1-15
4 Ex. 33—34; Matt. 19:16-30
5 Ex. 35—36; Matt. 20:1-16
6 Ex. 37—38; Matt. 20:17-34
7 Ex. 39—40; Matt. 21:1-22
8 Lev. 1—3; Matt. 21:23-46
9 Lev. 4—5; Matt. 22:1-14
10 Lev. 6—8; Matt. 22:15-46
11 Lev. 9—10; Matt. 23
12 Lev. 11—13; Matt. 24:1-31
13 Lev. 14—15; Matt. 24:32-51
14 Lev. 16—18; Matt. 25:1-30
15 Lev. 19—20; Matt. 25:31-46
16 Lev. 21—23; Matt. 26:1-35
17 Lev. 24—25; Matt. 26:36-56
18 Lev. 26—27; Matt. 26:57-75
19 Num. 1—2; Matt. 27:1-31
20 Num. 3—4; Matt. 27:32-66
21 Num. 5—6; Matt. 28
22 Num. 7; Mark 1:1-15
23 Num. 8—10; Mark 1:16-45
24 Num. 11—12; Mark 2:1-13
25 Num. 13—14; Mark 2:14-28
26 Num. 15—16; Mark 3:1-12
27 Num. 17—18; Mark 3:13-35
28 Num. 19—20; Mark 4:1-20
29 Num. 21; Mark 4:21-41
(If Feb. has 28 days, read 28-29.)

MARCH
1 Num. 22—24; Mark 5:1-20
2 Num. 25—26; Mark 5:21-43
3 Num. 27—29; Mark 6:1-13
4 Num. 30—31; Mark 6:14-32
5 Num. 32—33; Mark 6:33-56
6 Num. 34—36; Mark 7:1-23
7 Deut. 1—2; Mark 7:24-37
8 Deut. 3—4; Mark 8:1-10
9 Deut. 5—6; Mark 8:11-26
10 Deut. 7—9; Mark 8:27-38
11 Deut. 10—11; Mark 9:1-13
12 Deut. 12—14; Mark 9:14-29

13 Deut. 15—17; Mark 9:30-50
14 Deut. 18—20; Mark 10:1-16
15 Deut. 21—23; Mark 10:17-31
16 Deut. 24—26; Mark 10:32-52
17 Deut. 27—28; Mark 11:1-11
18 Deut. 29—30; Mark 11:12-33
19 Deut. 31—32; Mark 12:1-12
20 Deut. 33—34; Mark 12:13-27
21 Josh. 1—2; Mark 12:28-44
22 Josh. 3—4; Mark 13:1-13
23 Josh. 5—6; Mark 13:14-37
24 Josh. 7—8; Mark 14:1-11
25 Josh. 9—10; Mark 14:12-31
26 Josh. 11—12; Mark 14:32-52
27 Josh. 13—15; Mark 14:53-72
28 Josh. 16—18; Mark 15:1-15
29 Josh. 19—20; Mark 15:16-39
30 Josh. 21—22; Mark 15:40-47
31 Josh. 23—24; Mark 16

APRIL
1 Judg. 1—3; Luke 1:1-25
2 Judg. 4—5; Luke 1:26-38
3 Judg. 6; Luke 1:39-56
4 Judg. 7—8; Luke 1:57-80
5 Judg. 9; Luke 2:1-20
6 Judg. 10—12; Luke 2:21-40
7 Judg. 13—15; Luke 2:41-52
8 Judg. 16; Luke 3:1-20
9 Judg. 17—18; Luke 3:21-38
10 Judg. 19—20; Luke 4:1-13
11 Judg. 21; Luke 4:14-32
12 Ruth 1—2; Luke 4:33-44
13 Ruth 3—4; Luke 5:1-26
14 1 Sam. 1—2; Luke 5:27-39
15 1 Sam. 3—4; Luke 6:1-11
16 1 Sam. 5—6; Luke 6:12-49
17 1 Sam. 7—8; Luke 7:1-17
18 1 Sam. 9—10; Luke 7:18-35
19 1 Sam. 11—13; Luke 7:36-50
20 1 Sam. 14—15; Luke 8:1-18
21 1 Sam. 16—17; Luke 8:19-39
22 1 Sam. 18—19; Luke 8:40-56
23 1 Sam. 20—21; Luke 9:1-17
24 1 Sam. 22—23; Luke 9:18-45
25 1 Sam. 24—25; Luke 9:46-62
26 1 Sam. 26—27; Luke 10:1-24
27 1 Sam. 28—29; Luke 10:25-42
28 1 Sam. 30—31; Luke 11:1-13
29 2 Sam. 1—2; Luke 11:14-28
30 2 Sam. 3—4; Luke 11:29-54

MAY
1 2 Sam. 5—6; Luke 12:1-12
2 2 Sam. 7—8; Luke 12:13-34
3 2 Sam. 9—10; Luke 12:35-59
4 2 Sam. 11—12; Luke 13:1-17
5 2 Sam. 13—14; Luke 13:18-35
6 2 Sam. 15—16; Luke 14:1-24
7 2 Sam. 17—18; Luke 14:25-35
8 2 Sam. 19—20; Luke 15
9 2 Sam. 21—22; Luke 16:1-18
10 2 Sam. 23—24; Luke 16:19-31
11 1 Kings 1—2; Luke 17:1-19
12 1 Kings 3—4; Luke 17:20-37
13 1 Kings 5—6; Luke 18:1-17
14 1 Kings 7—8; Luke 18:18-43
15 1 Kings 9—11; Luke 19:1-27
16 1 Kings 12—13; Luke 19:28-48
17 1 Kings 14—15; Luke 20:1-26
18 1 Kings 16—17; Luke 20:27-47
19 1 Kings 18—19; Luke 21:1-28
20 1 Kings 20—21; Luke 21:29-38
21 1 Kings 22; Luke 22:1-23
22 2 Kings 1—3; Luke 22:24-53
23 2 Kings 4—5; Luke 22:54-71
24 2 Kings 6—7; Luke 23:1-12
25 2 Kings 8—9; Luke 23:13-32

26 2 Kings 10—11; Luke 23:33-56
27 2 Kings 12—13; Luke 24:1-12
28 2 Kings 14—15; Luke 24:13-53
29 2 Kings 16—17; John 1:1-18
30 2 Kings 18—20; John 1:19-51
31 2 Kings 21—23; John 2

JUNE
1 2 Kings 24—25; John 3:1-21
2 1 Chron. 1—2; John 3:22-36
3 1 Chron. 3—4; John 4:1-42
4 1 Chron. 5—6; John 4:43-54
5 1 Chron. 7—8; John 5:1-17
6 1 Chron. 9—10; John 5:18-47
7 1 Chron. 11—12; John 6:1-15
8 1 Chron. 13—15; John 6:16-40
9 1 Chron. 16—17; John 6:41-71
10 1 Chron. 18—19; John 7:1-36
11 1 Chron. 20—21; John 7:37-53
12 1 Chron. 22—24; John 8:1-11
13 1 Chron. 25—27; John 8:12-59
14 1 Chron. 28—29; John 9
15 2 Chron. 1—2; John 10:1-21
16 2 Chron. 3—4; John 10:22-42
17 2 Chron. 5—6; John 11
18 2 Chron. 7—9; John 12:1-19
19 2 Chron. 10—12; John 12:20-50
20 2 Chron. 13—16; John 13
21 2 Chron. 17—19; John 14
22 2 Chron. 20—21; John 15
23 2 Chron. 22—23; John 16
24 2 Chron. 24—25; John 17
25 2 Chron. 26—27; John 18
26 2 Chron. 28—29; John 19:1-16
27 2 Chron. 30—31; John 19:17-42
28 2 Chron. 32; John 20:1-18
29 2 Chron. 33—34; John 20:19-31
30 2 Chron. 35—36; John 21

JULY
1 Ezra 1—2; Acts 1
2 Ezra 3—4; Acts 2
3 Ezra 5—6; Acts 3
4 Ezra 7—8; Acts 4:1-22
5 Ezra 9—10; Acts 4:23-37
6 Neh. 1—3; Acts 5
7 Neh. 4—6; Acts 6
8 Neh. 7—9; Acts 7
9 Neh. 10—11; Acts 8:1-25
10 Neh. 12—13; Acts 8:26-40
11 Esth. 1—2; Acts 9:1-22
12 Esth. 3—6; Acts 9:23-43
13 Esth. 7—10; Acts 10:1-23
14 Job 1—3; Acts 10:24-48
15 Job 4—7; Acts 11
16 Job 8—10; Acts 12
17 Job 11—14; Acts 13:1-13
18 Job 15—17; Acts 13:14-52
19 Job 18—21; Acts 14
20 Job 22—24; Acts 15
21 Job 25—28; Acts 16:1-15
22 Job 29—31; Acts 16:16-40
23 Job 32—34; Acts 17:1-15
24 Job 35—37; Acts 17:16-34
25 Job 38—39; Acts 18
26 Job 40—42; Acts 19:1-20
27 Ps. 1—6; Acts 19:21-41
28 Ps. 7—12; Acts 20:1-16
29 Ps. 13—18; Acts 20:17-38
30 Ps. 19—24; Acts 21:1-16
31 Ps. 25—30; Acts 21:17-40

AUGUST
1 Ps. 31—36; Acts 22
2 Ps. 37—41; Acts 23
3 Ps. 42—47; Acts 24
4 Ps. 48—53; Acts 25
5 Ps. 54—58; Acts 26

6 Ps. 59—64; Acts 27
7 Ps. 65—68; Acts 28:1-15
8 Ps. 69—72; Acts 28:16-31
9 Ps. 73—77; Rom. 1:1-17
10 Ps. 78—80; Rom. 1:18-32
11 Ps. 81—86; Rom. 2
12 Ps. 87—89; Rom. 3
13 Ps. 90—95; Rom. 4
14 Ps. 96—102; Rom. 5
15 Ps. 103—106; Rom. 6
16 Ps. 107—111; Rom. 7
17 Ps. 112—118; Rom. 8:1-17
18 Ps. 119:1-88; Rom. 8:18-39
19 Ps. 119:89-176; Rom. 9
20 Ps. 120—129; Rom. 10
21 Ps. 130—136; Rom. 11
22 Ps. 137—140; Rom. 12
23 Ps. 141—145; Rom. 13
24 Ps. 146—150; Rom. 14
25 Prov. 1—3; Rom. 15
26 Prov. 4—6; Rom. 16
27 Prov. 7—9; 1 Cor. 1
28 Prov. 10—12; 1 Cor. 2
29 Prov. 13—14; 1 Cor. 3
30 Prov. 15—17; 1 Cor. 4
31 Prov. 18—20; 1 Cor. 5

SEPTEMBER
1 Prov. 21—23; 1 Cor. 6
2 Prov. 24—26; 1 Cor. 7
3 Prov. 27—29; 1 Cor. 8
4 Prov. 30—31; 1 Cor. 9
5 Ecd. 1—3; 1 Cor. 10
6 Ecd. 4—7; 1 Cor. 11
7 Ecd. 8—12; 1 Cor. 12
8 Song of Sol. 1—4; 1 Cor. 13
9 Song of Sol. 5—8; 1 Cor. 14
10 Isa. 1—4; 1 Cor. 15
11 Isa. 5—7; 1 Cor. 16
12 Isa. 8—9; 2 Cor. 1
13 Isa. 10—12; 2 Cor. 2
14 Isa. 13—14; 2 Cor. 3
15 Isa. 15—18; 2 Cor. 4
16 Isa. 19—22; 2 Cor. 5
17 Isa. 23—25; 2 Cor. 6
18 Isa. 26—29; 2 Cor. 7
19 Isa. 30—32; 2 Cor. 8
20 Isa. 33—35; 2 Cor. 9
21 Isa. 36—39; 2 Cor. 10
22 Isa. 40—41; 2 Cor. 11
23 Isa. 42—43; 2 Cor. 12
24 Isa. 44—47; 2 Cor. 13
25 Isa. 48—50; Gal. 1
26 Isa. 51—53; Gal. 2
27 Isa. 54—57; Gal. 3
28 Isa. 58—60; Gal. 4
29 Isa. 61—63; Gal. 5
30 Isa. 64—66; Gal. 6

OCTOBER
1 Jer. 1; Eph. 1
2 Jer. 2; Eph. 2
3 Jer. 3—4; Eph. 3
4 Jer. 5—6; Eph. 4
5 Jer. 7—8; Eph. 5
6 Jer. 9—10; Eph. 6
7 Jer. 11—12; Phil. 1
8 Jer. 13—14; Phil. 2
9 Jer. 15—17; Phil. 3
10 Jer. 18—19; Phil. 4
11 Jer. 20—21; Col. 1
12 Jer. 22—23; Col. 2
13 Jer. 24—25; Col. 3
14 Jer. 26; Col. 4
15 Jer. 27—28; 1 Thess. 1
16 Jer. 29—30; 1 Thess. 2
17 Jer. 31; 1 Thess. 3
18 Jer. 32; 1 Thess. 4

19 Jer. 33—34; 1 Thess. 5
20 Jer. 35—36; 2 Thess. 1
21 Jer. 37—38; 2 Thess. 2
22 Jer. 39—41; 2 Thess. 3
23 Jer. 42—43; 1 Tim. 1
24 Jer. 44—45; 1 Tim. 2
25 Jer. 46—47; 1 Tim. 3
26 Jer. 48; 1 Tim. 4
27 Jer. 49; 1 Tim. 5
28 Jer. 50; 1 Tim. 6
29 Jer. 51; 2 Tim. 1
30 Jer. 52; 2 Tim. 2
31 Lam. 1; 2 Tim. 3

NOVEMBER
1 Lam. 2; 2 Tim. 4
2 Lam. 3; Titus 1
3 Lam. 4; Titus 2
4 Lam. 5; Titus 3
5 Ezek. 1—2; Philem.
6 Ezek. 3—5; Heb. 1
7 Ezek. 6—7; Heb. 2
8 Ezek. 8—10; Heb. 3
9 Ezek. 11—12; Heb. 4
10 Ezek. 13—14; Heb. 5
11 Ezek. 15—16; Heb. 6
12 Ezek. 17—18; Heb. 7
13 Ezek. 19—20; Heb. 8
14 Ezek. 21—22; Heb. 9
15 Ezek. 23—24; Heb. 10
16 Ezek. 25—26; Heb. 11
17 Ezek. 27—28; Heb. 12
18 Ezek. 29—30; Heb. 13
19 Ezek. 31—32; Jas. 1
20 Ezek. 33—34; Jas. 2
21 Ezek. 35—37; Jas. 3
22 Ezek. 38—39; Jas. 4
23 Ezek. 40—41; Jas. 5
24 Ezek. 42—43; 1 Pet. 1
25 Ezek. 44—46; 1 Pet. 2
26 Ezek. 47—48; 1 Pet. 3
27 Dan. 1; 1 Pet. 4
28 Dan. 2; 1 Pet. 5
29 Dan. 3; 2 Pet. 1
30 Dan. 4; 2 Pet. 2

DECEMBER
1 Dan. 5—6; 2 Pet. 3
2 Dan. 7—8; 1 John 1
3 Dan. 9; 1 John 2
4 Dan. 10—12; 1 John 3
5 Hos. 1—3; 1 John 4
6 Hos. 4—6; 1 John 5
7 Hos. 7—8; 2 John
8 Hos. 9—10; 3 John
9 Hos. 11—12; Jude
10 Hos. 13—14; Rev. 1
11 Joel 1—3; Rev. 2
12 Amos 1—2; Rev. 3
13 Amos 3—4; Rev. 4
14 Amos 5—7; Rev. 5
15 Amos 8—9; Rev. 6
16 Obad.; Rev. 7
17 Jonah 1—4; Rev. 8
18 Mic. 1—2; Rev. 9
19 Mic. 3—4; Rev. 10
20 Mic. 5—7; Rev. 11
21 Nah. 1—3; Rev. 12
22 Hab. 1—3; Rev. 13
23 Zeph. 1—3; Rev. 14
24 Hag. 1—2; Rev. 15
25 Zech. 1—3; Rev. 16
26 Zech. 4—5; Rev. 17
27 Zech. 6—8; Rev. 18
28 Zech. 9—11; Rev. 19
29 Zech. 12—14; Rev. 20
30 Mal. 1—2; Rev. 21
31 Mal. 3—4; Rev. 22

BEHAVIOR & EMOTION IN WEIGHT MANAGEMENT

Learning what is healthy and what it takes physiologically to lose or manage weight will help only if you can cope with behavioral issues that arise.

Behavior Modification for Lifelong Weight Management

Practicing consistency and awareness are keys to success.

Meals

- Practice portion control. Eat slowly; chew food well.
- Avoid eating while watching TV or reading.
- Schedule your eating to help you eat less and focus more.
- Use a smaller plate; do not clean your plate; throw away leftover food immediately.
- Minimize contact—put food away after preparing a sandwich.
- Keep healthy snacks in sight and high calorie foods out of sight.
- Plan ahead for meals, snacks, and special events.

Shopping

- Shop on a full stomach.
- Shop from a list and buy foods that require preparation.
- Shop the outside aisles.

Eating Out

Thirty percent of meals eaten in the United States are eaten outside of the home; portions are often twice normal size.

- Help choose the restaurant.
- Order à la carte the same types of healthy food you would cook at home.
- Order first so you won't be influenced by others. Use breadbasket cautiously.
- Avoid alcohol.
- Ask for lowfat dressings on the side.
- Order grilled or broiled vegetables and meats.
- Exercise portion control. The average palm equals a three-ounce serving of meat; the end section of your thumb is about a tablespoon, and the end section of your little finger equals a teaspoon. Save half of your food for later.

Substitution Activities

- Walk instead of snacking and watching television.
- Perform activities not compatible with eating. Visit a neighbor, play a board game, write a letter, brush your teeth.
- Take a relaxing bath instead of bedtime snack.

Rewards

- Short-term: praise, money, new wardrobe, fantasy vacation
- Long-term: reduced body fat, cholesterol, blood pressure; increased energy

Develop a Healthy Body Image

- Get accustomed to looking at your body.
- Stop comparing yourself with others, especially "unreal" people in advertising.
- Focus on your body as a gift from God.

LITTLE CHANGES—BIG CALORIE DEFICIT

Little Change	Daily Caloric Impact	Yearly Caloric Impact	Annual Weight Loss
Substitute skim for 2% milk (2c/day)	60	21,900	6.3
Substitute reduced fat cheddar for regular (3-4 oz./week)	15	5,475	1.6
Substitute 2 egg whites for whole egg (3 eggs/week)	19	6,935	2.0
Substitute nonfat frozen yogurt for regular ice cream (3x/week)	21.4	7,821	2.2
Eat one less donut per week	29	10,429	3.0
Substitute reduced fat salad dressing for regular 3x/week	21.4	7,821	2.2
Eliminate one 12 oz. sugar sweetened soda/day	240	87,600	25.0
Walk one minute after each meal	12	4,380	1.3
Walk 10 extra minutes/day*	40	14,600	4.2
Walk 15 extra minutes/day (one mile)*	60	21,900	6.3

Chart by Julie Opp using nutrition facts food labels (cheese, milk, salad dressings).
Walking calculations adapted from Eleanor Noss Whitney and Sharon Rady Rolfes,
Understanding Nutrition, 7th edition (St. Paul: West Publishing, Co., 1996), 284.
*assuming 100 calories burned per mile (average burned by 150 lb. person walking 4.0 miles/hr)

STRENGTH TRAINING TIPS

1. Start Out Slowly—Staying light on resistance and taking time to learn proper form and technique will help keep you injury free and minimize soreness.
2. Go Large to Small—Beginners should design their exercise routine to work the larger muscle groups of the hips, legs, and torso first; then move to the smaller muscle groups of the arms, waist, and lower back.
3. Progress Systematically—When your muscles adapt to the resistance, increase it! For example, if you're working at 12 RM, once you can get 13 reps in proper form, increase your next workout's weight by approximately 5 percent.
4. Lift With Control—Too often, folks end up jerking the resistance around and lifting momentum! Make it a habit to lift smoothly. Lift on about a two second count and lower on a four second count to provide better results.
5. Range of Motion—Strive to work the muscle through its normal full range of motion. Avoid restricted movements which have limited value and may lead to reduction in joint mobility.
6. Mix It Up—Vary one or two routines at least every four to six weeks. You can manipulate things such as the resistance load, the exercises performed, number of repetitions, number of sets, and length of rest periods.
7. Keep Records—Keeping accurate records will allow you to see workout-by-workout progress. Your record should list the exercises, date, resistance, repetitions, and total training time as a minimum.
8. Don't Under-Train—Strive to work all major muscle groups in the body at least two days per week. Try not to allow more than 96 hours between workouts.
9. Don't Over-Train—Allow muscle groups at least 48-72 hours of recovery time between strength-training bouts. Never strength train the same muscle groups two days in a row. Get adequate rest and proper nutrition.
10. Buddy Up—As you progress, particularly in free weights, a workout partner can offer encouragement and added safety through spotting.

How quickly will I see results?

Initial training status plays an important role in how quickly one will see results. Untrained individuals (those with no resistance training experience or those who have not trained in several years) will respond quickly to initial training. One will show a rapid increase in muscular strength long before visual changes in muscle size are seen. Review of the literature reveals that muscular strength increases approximately 40 percent in the first four to eight weeks of training.

Which is better, machines or free-weights?

Both machines and free weights have their advantages and disadvantages. It is important to select the mode of exercise based on your individual needs, goals, initial abilities, and preference. Beginners tend to do better starting with predominantly machines. Machines require less technique and are safer. More advanced weight trainers will benefit from the variety offered through free weights and functional movements that mimic everyday activities. Don't get so hung up on finding the best mode of training that you become paralyzed! As long as you provide overload and progression you will increase your strength no matter what kind of resistance you choose.

TOTAL BODY BASIC STRENGTH TRAINING ROUTINE

See week 4 for specific information on strength training and implementing these exercises into your exercise plan. Below are descriptions of the exercises on page 39.

1. Squats. This exercise uses the quadriceps, hamstrings and gluteus muscles. Stand with feet shoulder width apart and hands on waist. Bend knees and squat down as if you were sitting in a chair. Hold for a slow count of two. Press through feet and return to standing. Keep back straight and abdominals tight. Do not allow knees to extend past your toes.

2. Lunges. This exercise uses the quadriceps, hamstrings and gluteus muscles. Take one giant step forward keeping torso centered between legs. Raise heel on back foot so weight is distributed between the ball of the back foot and the heel of the front foot. Keep abdominals tight. You should feel a slight stretching across the hip of the back leg. Use a wall or chair to assist with balance if necessary. Keep spine straight as you bend both knees and lunge down. Avoid moving forward or backward. Do not allow knee to touch the floor. Contract the muscles of your legs and buttocks and press up to the starting position.

3. Calf Raises. This exercise uses the Gastrocnemius and Soleus muscles of the lower leg. Stand with front of foot on the edge of a stair or raised platform and your heels hanging off and slightly lower than the step. Hold a wall or other structure for balance. Slowly press up onto your toes raising your heels and contracting the muscles of your calves. Slowly lower your heels lower than the step you are standing on to return to starting position.

4. Chest Press. This exercise uses the Pectoralis major and minor muscles and the triceps. Lie down on the bench with feet on the floor. Keep abdominals tight to support spine through the lift. Wrap tubing under the bench to create resistance and tension in the tubing. Hold ends of tubing in each hand with elbows out from your sides, even or just slightly below shoulder level, and bent 90 degrees. Press hands toward the ceiling and allow hands to touch above the chest. Arms should be straight but not fully extended at the elbow. Keep chest lifted through the range of motion. Slowly return to starting position and feel a slight stretch across the chest.

5. Seated Row. This exercise uses the rhomboids, latissimus dorsi, and the biceps. Sit on the edge of a chair with your legs extended and heels on the floor. Place tubing around feet and point toes away from body. Grasp handles. If using weights, hold weights in same position as handles of tubing. Keeping shoulder pressed down, row elbows back and hands to the ribs. Squeeze the middle back muscles and hold for a slow count of 2. Avoid leaning back as you row. Use abdominal muscles to stabilize torso through the range of motion. Slowly return to starting position allowing shoulders to slightly round but do not lean forward.

6. Shoulder Shrug. This exercise uses the trapezius muscle. Stand in the center of the tubing with both feet. Grasp the handles with arms fully extended at sides. Using the muscles of your shoulders and upper back, shrug shoulders up toward the ears. Slowly return to starting position.

7. Lateral Raises. This exercise uses the deltoids. Stand on one end of the tubing and grasp one handle. Create tension in the tubing by decreasing the amount of tubing between the handle and foot. Slowly lift arm to the side until the arm is shoulder height. Keep the elbow slightly bent. Slowly return to the starting position. Repeat on the other arm.

8. Triceps Dips with a chair. This exercise uses the triceps. Sit on the edge of a chair. Place your hands on the seat of the chair next to your body letting your fingers curl over the edge of the chair. With feet on the floor, move body off of chair supporting body weight on your arms and feet. Bend elbows and lower body down until elbows are at a 90-degree angle. Press through the hands contracting the triceps and press body back up to starting position. Keep back straight through motion. If you experience pain in your shoulders stop the exercise.

9. Biceps Curls. This exercise strengthens the biceps. Stand on the tubing with your feet shoulder width apart and your knees slightly bent for support. Hold tubing handles in each hand with your palms-up grip. Slowly curl the hands up toward your shoulder. Pause, then slowly lower to the starting position. Keep elbows stationary during the curl.

10. Abdominal Crunches. This exercise strengthens the abdominals. Lie on your back with your feet resting flat on the floor, your knees bent at a 90-degree angle, your hands cupping your ears and your elbows out to the sides. Tilt your pelvis slightly to flatten your back against the floor. Contract your abs and slowly lift your shoulders and head off the floor about 30 degrees. Hold for two seconds, then lower them back to the starting position. Do not pull on your neck during the exercise. To avoid neck strain, keep your chin forward (you should always be able to fit a fist between your chin and your chest) and your eyes facing the ceiling.

11. Back Extensions. This exercises uses the erector spinea and lumbar muscles in the lower back. Lie face down on an exercise mat or towel. Place hands under chin with palms down. Using the muscles of your lower back and gluteals, slowly lift your upper body off the floor. Exhale as you lift. Hold the lift for a slow count of 2. Keep your head in alignment with your spine. Lift only until you feel a slight contraction in your lower back. If you have challenges or pain in your lower back, ask your doctor or physical therapist if this exercise is acceptable for you.

COGNITIVE DISTORTIONS

All or Nothing. Self-evaluation of life as black or white. Interpreting one mistake as total failure or complete stupidity. Example: "I always pick the slow line." or "I'll never amount to anything."

Overgeneralization. All-or-nothing thinking; stereotyping; interpreting one example as an unbreakable pattern. Example: One friend gossips about you; you conclude no one can be trusted. "All women are …" "All churches do …"

Mental Filter. Dwelling on negative details exclusively. Example: You make a presentation to a hundred people, and one person questions your data. You conclude that your work was wasted and that you looked foolish presenting it.

Disqualifying. Rejecting positive experiences by self-deprecation or self-effacement. Example: You're complimented for an innovative idea and respond, "Anyone could have come up with that; he's just being nice." The language of "Yes, but …"

Jumping to Conclusions. Relying on mind reading to interpret life. Example: You see a friend in the distance who doesn't acknowledge your wave, so you conclude she no longer likes you. Or, predicting future outcomes as the basis for your words or actions. Example: "There's no point in asking my brother for help; he'll just say no."

Magnification. Catastrophizing the effect of a mistake or negative event. Example: Being unavoidably caught in traffic, you conclude you'll be fired and your desk already cleaned out by the time you arrive.

Minimization. Inappropriately shrinking positive personal qualities or events until they appear trivial. Examples: "So what if we're expecting; it doesn't take any talent to get pregnant." "Big deal if I yell at my kids; they know I love them."

MOANS Statements. Unproductive use of words *must, ought, always, never,* and especially *should.* These words create feelings of being pressured, inadequacy, incompetence. Example: "You never care about anyone but yourself."

Labeling and Mislabeling. Overly simplistic thinking about complex thoughts, emotions, and actions. Examples: "She's a Lanford; they all act that way." "He's just a bureaucratic flunkie—they never care." "I'm just a fat slob."

Personalization. Also known as "the mother of all guilt!" Even when something isn't your fault, you own the guilt for it. Example: Your child fails an exam and you say, "I'm such an awful parent."

Perfectionism—my personal favorite. The unrealistic expectation that you and others must be perfect all the time, and when that's not so, it is catastrophic. Example: "If that cake falls, I don't know what I'll do; it will be just awful." "My son is taking a semester off from college; that's just terrible." Perfectionism is an unusually cruel form of self-abuse, for it doesn't permit any form of success, satisfaction, or pleasure for who you are and what you do.[1]

When you become aware your thoughts are like those distortions, what do you do? A simple four-step process is described in *The Wellness Book:*[2]

1. STOP. Pull over, stop walking, take a break. Acknowledge perfectionistic, all-or-nothing thinking, and stop.

2. BREATHE. Take several slow, deep breaths—require your diaphragmatic muscle to fill and empty your lungs as you breathe in and out. That minute of slow breathing releases physical tension and begins to interrupt the automatic stress response. It also allows time and space to voice a prayer, as the apostle Paul encouraged his Philippian friends to do.

3. REFLECT. Intentionally, thoughtfully, challenge distorted thoughts or irrational beliefs. Ask yourself questions such as:
- Is this thought really true?
- Am I jumping to conclusions?
- Does it serve me well to think this way?
- Can I interpret this situation differently?
- Is the threat really as bad as I first thought?
- What's the worst that could happen?
- What proof do I have that I can't handle it?

4. CHOOSE. Now you're ready for an intentional response and not a knee-jerk reaction. Choose actions and words that allow you to recognize yourself in the midst of the stress and afterwards when the stress is resolved. So, choose creatively! The first three steps will enhance your ability to think differently, to be more objective about yourself, to quiet the emotions stirred up by those distorted ways of thinking.

[1]Adapted from David Burns, *Feeling Good: The New Mood Therapy* (New York: Avon Books, 1999), 42–43.
[2]Herbert Benson and Eileen M. Stuart, *The Wellness Book: The Comprehensive Guide to Maintaining Health and Treating Stress-Related Illness* (New York: Simon & Schuster, 1993), 237.

How to Become a Christian

One of our greatest satisfactions on earth is having a healthy body. When we feel sluggish or tired—or we have an ongoing medical condition—life simply does not work the way God intended. With sin came disease and death. We were created as spiritual beings with a capacity to know and love God. Because we were made to be like God, we have an empty spot in our lives until we find fulfillment in Him. In Jesus Christ, we find the hope, peace, and joy that is only possible through a personal relationship with God.

John 3:16 says, "'God so loved the world that he gave his one and only Son, that whoever believes in him shall not perish but have eternal life.'" In order to live our earthly lives "to the full" (see John 10:10), we must accept God's gift of love.

A relationship with God begins by admitting that we are not perfect and continue to fall short of God's standards. Romans 3:23 says, "All have sinned and fall short of the glory of God." The price for these wrongdoings is separation from God. We deserve to pay the price for our sin. "The wages (or price) of sin is death, but the gift of God is eternal life in Christ Jesus our Lord" (Rom. 6:23).

God's love comes to us right in the middle of our sin. "God demonstrates his own love for us in this: While we were still sinners, Christ died for us" (Rom. 5:8). He doesn't ask us to clean up our lives first—in fact, without His help, we are incapable of living by His standards. He wants us to come to Him as we are.

Forgiveness begins when we admit our sin to God. When we do, He is faithful to forgive and restore our relationship with Him. "If we confess our sins, he is faithful and just and will forgive us our sins and purify us from all unrighteousness" (1 John 1:9).

Scripture confirms that this love gift and relationship with God is not just for a special few, but for everyone. "'Everyone who calls on the name of the Lord will be saved'" (Rom. 10:13).

If you would like to receive God's gift of salvation, pray this prayer:

> *Dear God, I know that I am imperfect and separated from You. Please forgive me of my sin and adopt me as Your child. Thank You for this gift of life through the sacrifice of Your Son. I will live my life for You. Amen.*

If you prayed this prayer for the first time, you are now a child of God. In your Bible, read 1 John 5:11-12. This verse assures you that if you have accepted God's Son, Jesus Christ, as your Savior and Lord, you have this eternal life.

Share your experience with your *Fit 4* facilitator, someone in your group, your pastor, or a trusted Christian friend. Welcome to God's family!

Leader Guide

With All My Strength: God's Design for Physical Wellness is a continuing study in *Fit 4: A LifeWay Christian Wellness Plan*. This study is open to anyone who chooses to participate, whether or not the person has taken another *Fit 4* course or continuing study. Treat it as you would any one-hour group discipleship course.

Relationship to *Fit 4*

Review page 4 to understand how this study incorporates the basic principles of *Fit 4*.

Because this study emphasizes only one of four essential components of wellness, encourage participants to use the *Accountability Journal* provided with each member book to record daily food and exercise choices. Some participants may not have committed to the *Fit 4* Guidelines for Healthy Eating (see *Journal*, p. 20) or the *Fit 4* F.I.T.T. exercise model for developing a personalized exercise plan (see *Journal*, p. 14). Promote the concept of whole-person health by encouraging nutritional and fitness goals as an integral part of total wellness. The Professor Phitt suggestions each week offer practical application activities.

Introductory Session

Because of the *Fit 4* terminology used, as well as references to Professor Phitt and other *Fit 4* resources, we recommend that participants view the 15-minute *Fit 4* Introductory Session video found at the beginning of both the *Fitness* and *Nutrition* group session videos in the *Fit 4 Plan Kit* (ISBN 0-6330-0580-0). Preview the video and have it cued at the beginning of the tape. Arrange for a TV/VCR for the introductory session only. A lesson plan for the introductory session is found on page 104.

Sessions 1-10

Each week's reading assignment can be read in one sitting or spaced during the week. Encourage participants to memorize the Verse(s) to Know and say the Scripture together at the beginning of each session. Session plans for the 10 weeks are found on pages 104-111. They are guides to help you lead discussion.

Encourage participants to ask questions and make comments from their reading. The benefit to each participant will increase as he or she completes each lesson's margin

Lifestyle Discipline activities as well as the learning activities highlighted by the *Fit 4* logo. Calling attention to these elements of the lesson will promote their use. Otherwise, members may assume they are unimportant.

Leading the Wrap-Up Session

Session 11 (week 12 of the study) is the final session of each *Fit 4* continuing course. In this session, lead a time of sharing, reflection, planning for the future, and praying. Several ideas for informal closure activities are suggested on page 111. Review these a few weeks before session 11 so you can plan ahead. Include the class in the planning.

Your Role as Facilitator

Like other members of your group, you are on your own wellness journey. No one is looking to you as an expert on physical wellness. Your role is to guide the group experience using the session plans provided.

Before each session, arrive early. Provide a sign-up sheet at the door and name tags, if needed. Have on hand extra Bibles, pens or pencils, and member books for the first two sessions. Pray for each member, the group process, and yourself on a regular basis. Use the attendance sheet to note absentees; then contact them during the week.

Place chairs in a circle and sit with other members. Begin and end each session on time. Open and close the sessions with prayer. Encourage member discussion of the week's material. Avoid doing too much talking. Keep the discussion positive, in keeping with the emphasis on physical wellness. Avoid letting members get too personal or graphic in sharing.

Be aware of special needs in the class. If a class member is unsaved, be prepared to follow the leadership of the Holy Spirit to know the right time to talk to that person privately to lead them to Christ (see How to Become a Christian, p. 102). If other problems surface, be prepared to refer members to Christian counselors in the area.

After the session, complete your weekly reading assignment and your *Accountability Journal*. Learn each week's Verse(s) to Know. Follow the instructions in this Guide for planning for the next session.

INTRODUCTORY SESSION

Session Goals

To introduce participants to the concept of whole-person health and to enlist participation in this study.

Before the Session

- Set up the TV/VCR and cue the tape to the Introductory Session video.
- Arrange chairs so everyone can see the TV screen and each other.
- Supply name tags for each person.
- Provide an attendance sheet and pen.
- Have on hand one copy of the member book and *Accountability Journal* for every person expected.
- Before members arrive, pray for God's guidance.

During the Session

Greet members as they arrive. Have them sign the attendance sheet and give a phone number or email address. Instruct them to complete and wear the provided name tag. Open with prayer.

Introduce yourself and ask participants to share their names and one interesting fact about themselves. Distribute copies of *With All My Strength: God's Design for Physical Wellness* and the *Accountability Journal*.

Explain that although this study is open to anyone, it is a continuing study in *Fit 4: A LifeWay Christian Wellness Plan*. Say, During this session we will watch the *Fit 4* Introductory Session video to acquaint you with the concept of whole-person health and to introduce you to terms that will be used throughout the study. Ask members to turn to page 8 in their Member Books and write responses on the Viewer Guide as you play the Introductory Session video.

Ask volunteers to share responses to the Viewer Guide. Review pages 4 and 5 of the Member Book. Instruct participants to put their *Accountability Journals* in a three-ring binder. Highlight the information on pages 4-25. Explain that the *Accountability Journal* is a voluntary tool to encourage a wellness lifestyle. No one will evaluate their entries. Ask them to turn to page 27, circle tomorrow's day, and write the date. Encourage the group to begin tomorrow recording their food and exercise choices.

Overview week 1 by having participants turn through the pages as you talk about various sections. Explain the purpose of the Verses to Know and the margin activities. Point out that the material can be read in one sitting or by sections during the week. Call attention to page 8, which lists other *Fit 4* resources, such as the *fit4.com* Web site.

Allow time for participants to ask questions. Assign week 1. Collect payment for materials, if needed. Close the session with a word of encouragement and prayer.

SESSION 1

Session Goals

To encourage members to view physical health as a vital part of total wellness and a relationship with Christ as the starting point of the wellness journey.

Before the Session

- Provide name tags and a three-by-five-inch card for each member.
- Make four signs: EMOTIONS, MIND, SPIRIT, and BODY, one each page. Display at the front of the room.
- Be prepared to share the Plan of Salvation (p. 102).

During the Session

As members arrive, ask them to write their names on a name tag. Invite persons who were not present last session to briefly introduce themselves and share one interesting fact that few people would know about them. Allow 3-5 minutes for introductions.

Open the session with prayer. Distribute the three-by-five inch cards and ask members to write the Verses to Know from memory. Discuss how these verses remind us that we are total people. Invite members to share the physical challenge they thought of on page 9 of week 1. Refer to the words you displayed on the wall as members discuss this experience.

Briefly discuss how our physical condition is a ministry tool. Ask someone to share a physical ministry in which they participate.

On a white board, have members list various health fads. Ask, Have some of these fads passed? Are these healthy options? How are believers to respond to societal fads? Read 1 John 2:17. Emphasize the importance of doing the will of God over what the world encourages.

Review the "Total Wellness Assessment" (p. 89-95). Invite volunteers to share what they learned about themselves through this activity. Share your own observations.

Say, The wellness journey is not complete without a relationship with Christ. Share your personal salvation testimony and go through the Plan of Salvation on page 102 reviewing each point and Scripture. Invite participants to accept Him as personal Savior. Encourage members with questions to contact you after class for further discussion. Make assignments. Close the session by saying the prayer on page 102 or your own prayer.

Assignments for this Week:
- Complete Week 2 in your Member Workbook.
- Record food and activity in *Accountability Journal*.

After the Session
- Pray for the members of your class.
- Contact each member during the week to encourage and answer any questions.
- Read "Fit 4 Health Eating Guidelines" and "Fit 4 Food Guide" on pages 20-21 of the *Accountability Journal*.

SESSION 2

Session Goals
To provide members with sufficient information on weight management that they can develop a lifestyle eating and exercise plan that will continue for a lifetime.

Before the Session
- Locate a picture of a healthy, smiling baby to display at the next group session.
- Gather samples of low-fat, sugar free products; arrange them on a display table.

During the Session
As members arrive, ask them to wear a nametag. Display the picture of a healthy baby. Introduce the session goals. Say, Babies usually do not have weight problems (yet). The best way to avoid a problem is to never let it happen,

but it's never too late to develop a healthy eating plan. Pray, asking God to open our minds to His disciplines in our wellness journey.

Read together the Verse to Know on page 17 and share the definition of the word *discipline* in the margin. Briefly discuss the statistics given in the American Profile on page 17. Ask someone to read the two reasons given on pages 17-18. Allow time for members to relate their ideas on how Calories In (p. 20) and Calories Out (pp. 18-19) can alter these reasons for obesity.

Discuss the American Heart Association Guidelines (pp. 21-22). Ask someone to read Proverbs 4:13. Talk about the displayed samples of healthy foods.

Form groups to discuss healthy food plans vs. commercial weight loss programs (6-8 minutes). Ask each group to share ideas. Then emphasize that the goal is developing eating habits that last a lifetime.

Read the definition of management in the first paragraph of page 17. Discuss the core requirement of true motivation and the elements of successful weight management on page 24. Emphasize positive outlook and patience.

Make assignments. Give a brief introduction to week 3. Enlist someone to read aloud Psalm 139:1-3. Share prayer requests. Close with prayer.

Assignments for this Week:
- Complete week 3 in Member Workbook.
- Record food and activity in *Accountability Journal*.
- Complete the Body Mass Index calculation on page 19 of the *Accountability Journal*.

After the Session
- Pray for the members of your class.
- Contact each member during the week to encourage and answer any questions.

SESSION 3

Session Goals
To understand the advantages and disadvantages of vitamin, mineral, and herb supplements used in our diets.

Before the Session

- Write these scriptures on three-by-five-inch cards: Matthew 6:19-21; Matthew 6:25-26; Matthew 6:33; Psalm 139:14-16; Matthew 10:30; Luke 12:7.
- Option: Locate a picture of a strong person or well developed weight lifter to create interest in Week 4.

During the Session

Read together the Verse to Know and pray, thanking God for His blessings. Enlist one member to read Professor Phitt's comments on page 25. Allow 6-8 minutes for members to plan a daily menu using the serving numbers and items listed in paragraph two (p. 25). Ask volunteers to share their menus.

Distribute Scripture cards and ask the member with Matthew 6:19-21 to read it. Refer to UPREACH on page 27 and discuss how reading and meditating on God's Word can be a strong antioxidant for spiritual rust spots. Refer to the antioxidant chart on page 28 and ask members to circle at least three new food sources that they will include in their menu planning.

Have members read the remaining Scriptures in the order given above, and encourage volunteers to share the results of the activity on pages 29-30.

Invite personal testimonies on the pros and cons of herbs. Emphasis that you should ALWAYS check with your doctor before taking any new vitamin or herbal supplement. NEVER take anything without reading the information given with/on the bottle. Stress OUTREACH on page 30. Read Proverbs 23:20-21 and 25:16 and ask members to include these warnings in their outreach.

Allow time for participants to ask questions. Overview week 4 to maintain interest. (Suggestion: Show a picture of a strong person or well-developed weight lifter.) Make assignments. Take prayer requests. Ask a volunteer to pray. Close by reading together Mark 12:30-32.

Assignments for this Week:

- Complete Week 4 in Member Workbook.
- Record food and activity in *Accountability Journal*.
- Complete the "Physical Activity Readiness Questionnaire" on page 12 of the *Accountability Journal*.

After the Session

- Pray for the members of your class.
- Contact your class, telling them about the special guest in next week's class.

SESSION 4

Session Goals

To help class members further understand the concepts and benefits of strength training; to apply spiritual, emotional, and mental strength training concepts.

Before the Session

- Invite a local fitness professional to session 4 to discuss strength training. If you have such a person in your church, utilize him or her. If not, contact a local gym, health club, physical education or athletic department at a college or university, or a coach from a high school. Give the person chapter 4 so he/she is familiar with the material. Ask the person to speak 30-35 minutes.
- Gather information about local gyms and health clubs that are available for members. Discover free opportunities for exercise in your community. Provide this information to the class as a handout.

During the Session

As members arrive, invite them to discuss what they learned from this week's chapter on strength training. If you have a fitness professional as a guest in your class, introduce this person. Open the session with prayer.

Allow the guest 30-35 minutes to discuss strength training and answer questions from the class. Then, have the members recite the Verse to Know from page 33. Explain that God, our healer, helps us reap the benefits of strength and better health. Ask for prayer requests and close the session in prayer, remembering these requests.

If you do not have a guest, open with prayer and begin class by discussing the strength training terms from pages 34-35. Discuss the principals of program design highlighting the need to challenge our muscles to continually adapt to new weights as we get stronger.

Have someone read the OUTREACH activity on page 35. Discuss ideas for everyday random acts of kindness.

How do these acts of kindness reflect Christ to others? Allow for testimonies from those who have performed such acts this week. Encourage members to seek opportunities to help others without expecting a return.

Have the class recall the story of Samson (Judg. 16:4-22). Discuss the advantages and disadvantages of Samson's strength. What caused Samson to lose his strength? (He disobeyed God and allowed his hair to be cut.) How did Samson's disobedience effect him mentally, emotionally, spiritually and physically? Stress that when we obey God we reap benefits in all areas.

Remind members to complete the UPREACH activity on page 33 and seek medical consultation if necessary. Make assignments. Ask for prayer requests and close the session with prayer, remembering the requests.

Assignments for this Week:
- Complete Week 5 in Member Workbook.
- Record food and activity in *Accountability Journal*.
- Complete the "Calculate Your Target Heart Rate" form on page 18 of the *Accountability Journal*.
- Read "F.I.T.T. Principles" in the *Accountability Journal* on pages 14-15.

After the Session
- Pray for the members of your class.
- Complete your study of week 5.

SESSION 5

Session Goals
To discuss the various fitness options available; to encourage members to find an activity they enjoy and will use to improve fitness.

Before the Session
- Gather photos of various fitness options featured in week 5. In addition, find one picture of a person sitting doing nothing. Look in the newspaper, magazines, in personal photos, or on the Internet for options. Display the pictures.

During the Session
Open the session with prayer thanking God for our professions and the mental, emotional, physical and spiritual strength to complete these tasks.

Introduce this week's lesson by allowing each person to share their chosen profession. Ask each person to determine on a scale of 1 to 10 (1 being none at all and 10 being constantly), how much movement and physically challenging activity their daily job requires. Then have members share their estimated level of physical activity.

Point to the pictures of various fitness options displayed around the room. Ask members to stand by the picture that best demonstrates the fitness option in which they most often participate. Have volunteers share why they like that activity. Then have members move to an activity they don't currently choose but would like to try. Encourage members to try new activities to reduce boredom and use different muscles.

Have members return to their seats and turn to the Energy Expenditure chart on page 47. Explain that we take in energy whenever we eat. Food is the fuel for our activities. Review the chart comparing the sedentary activities and the active options. Have members put a check by 3 active things they will do next week.

Have the class say the Verse to Know from page 41. Ask, What does it mean to "walk in the light?" Is this a physical, mental, emotional or spiritual activity? (Answer: All, because we are whole people.) Say, When we walk in the Light we are fellowshipping with God, and this fellowship will help change our thinking, balance our emotions, strengthen our souls, and benefit our bodies. How do you know you are walking in the light? Have a class member read 1 John 2:3 for the answer.

Encourage the class to record their activities and exercise in the *Accountability Journal*. Remind them that recording their progress helps them know if they are on target.

Overview week 6 to maintain interest. Ask for prayer requests. Invite a volunteer to close the session in prayer remembering the mentioned requests.

Assignments for this Week:
- Complete Week 6 in Member Workbook.
- Record food and activity in *Accountability Journal*.

After the Session
- Pray for the members of your class.

SESSION 6
Session Goals
To discuss the characteristics of eating and exercise disorders and understand its addictive qualities. Members will also discover the spiritual "eating disorders" and how to avoid these in their walk with God.

Before the Session
- Visit the Web sites referenced in the chapter and print information on eating and exercise disorders that will benefit the class and add to discussion on the topic.
- Provide three-by-five inch cards for each class member.

During the Session
As members arrive, distribute three-by-five inch cards and ask them to write the Verse to Know from memory. Ask for prayer requests and say a prayer remembering these requests. Introduce the Eating Disorders topic.

Discuss Kelly Preston's struggle with anorexia. Ask, How did this disorder impact her physically, mentally, emotionally and spiritually?

Say, Eating disorders are not about food and/or weight. These are the symptoms of the disease, similar to how an alcoholic uses alcohol as a medication. While it is important that we learn the characteristics, consequences, treatments, and ways to help someone, it's just as important to realize the deeper control issues and how these disorders affect the entire person—physically, emotionally, mentally, and spiritually.

Give a review of the information you discovered on the Web sites referenced in the chapter.

Divide the class into two groups. Have one group discuss the characteristics of anorexia. Then instruct the group to draw spiritual comparisons for spiritual eating disorders, answering the question, How could a believer have

"spiritual anorexia"? (Sample answers may include: not "feeding on" or studying God's word, avoiding contact with other believers, allowing sin to slow their spiritual maturity, fearing a closer walk with God, obsessing with spiritual activities without a relationship to Christ.)

Ask group 2 to discuss the characteristics of bulimia and answer the question, How could a believer have "spiritual bulimia"? (Sample answers may include: taking in their spiritual food only on Sundays, living lives that aren't Christlike, isolating themselves from other believers, complaining and dissatisfaction with things at church, seeking spiritual fulfillment in resources other than God's Word and a relationship with Christ). After 5-7 minutes have each group report.

Ask, Can spiritual eating disorders be just as damaging as physical ones? (Yes) How? Allow the class time to respond.

Invite members to recite aloud the Verse to Know. Encourage them to apply this verse every day as they follow Christ.

Close the session with silent prayer allowing members to reflect on their own walk with Christ and renewing their commitment to follow Him each day. After a few minutes of silence, close with a spoken prayer.

Assignments for this Week:
- Complete Week 7 in Member Workbook.
- Record food and activity in *Accountability Journal*.
-

After the Session
- Pray for the members of your class
- Is any member falling behind in his/her reading? Contact this person and offer encouragement or assistance.

SESSION 7

Session Goal
To identify causes of stress and possible actions for relief to the mind, body and soul.

During the Session
Greet members and record attendance. Share prayer requests and enlist a volunteer to pray. Say the Verse to

Know together. Ask members to turn to page 57 and list their top five stressors in the margin. Ask, Do these circumstances help to fulfill Matthew 6:33? Read the session goal and Luke 12:22.

Discuss the Words to Know on pages 58-59 and ask volunteers to share examples of each. Ask, How do we get stressed? What stressors do you invite into your life? Discuss in detail the categories of stress and allow members to give examples of some of the stressors that can/can not be avoided; stress that can be modified; and stress that we create for ourselves. While this session is not a counseling session for the over-stressed, be alert to persons who might need help, encouragement, or referral to the pastor or a Christian counselor.

Emphasize that we do have choices. Call attention to the Stress Warning Signals on page 62 and ask, Are you stressed? Try the UPREACH activity; there is relief in time spent with our Heavenly Father. Remind members of How to Become a Christian on page 102 and allow time for responses.

Explain again: we do have choices. The battle is won or lost in the mind. What we think, we are. Discuss cognitive distortions on page 101 of the Appendix. Ask, How do these distortions lead to stress? End with the statement that our energy goes with our focus. Quote Philippians 4:13. Make assignments and close the session with prayer.

Assignments for this Week:
- Complete week 8 in Member Workbook.
- Record food and activity in *Accountability Journal*.

After the Session
- Pray for the members of your class.
- Send a note to encourage each person in your class.

SESSION 8

Session Goals
To dispel myths about aging and replace with truths that promote life-long habits that lead to successful aging.

Before the Session
- Provide paper and pencils for each class member.
- As members sign in, give them a piece of paper and ask each to put on it the age they classify as "old."

During the Session
Discuss briefly reasons for their opinions about "old." Read the session goal and pray that God will help us to realize that our days are numbered and we should maximize each to the fullest for His glory and honor.

Assign each of the six myths to a group or member to summarize the concepts in each. Keep discussion within two or three minutes for each myth and end each summary with the truth that exists.

Discuss the following questions:
- How can you avoid disease and disability?
- What can you do to maximize your cognitive fitness? your physical fitness?
- What does the phrase, "remain actively engaged in life" mean to you or to a senior you know? (The United States government recognizes 55 and older as Older Workers.)
- What are you doing to keep an attitude of life-long learning and spiritual growth?

Say, These are the key elements of successful aging given by Rowe and Kahn on page 68. Ask, When does the aging process begin? When is the right time to start life-long habits that will produce successful aging? (Now.)

Ask a volunteer to read Psalms 71:5-6,18, the mission statement for all seniors. Encourage members to record the scripture references in the last three pages of the chapter for future use in maintaining a positive faith in God and His will for the body and time He gives us.

Read together the Verse to Know as a class, encouraging members to memorize as a practice in cognitive strength building. Close with the thought: Age, though determined by the number of years you live, is really a state of mind. Pray thanking God that He is the One who has numbered our days.

Assignments for this Week:
- Complete Week 9 in Member Workbook.
- Record food and activity in *Accountability Journal*.

After the Session
- Pray for your class members.

SESSION 9

Session Goals
To compare lifestyle and genetic causes that impact diseases and health problems; to encourage members to change what can be changed.

Before the Session
- Prepare a poster containing the Serenity Prayer. (See the lesson plan below for the words to this prayer.)

During the Session
Read 1 Corinthians 10:11 and direct members to page 74. Ask them to silently answer the questions under What Do We Mean by "Lifestyle"? and silently pray that we will be receptive to what God is revealing about our lifestyle choices. After a minute or so, close the prayer time.

Read UPREACH on page 74. Emphasis that how we live and eat every day, and the genes we inherit from our parents make us who and what we are. Review and then discuss the key terms on cardiovascular disease on page 75. Encourage each member to commit to completing the INREACH activity and to knowing their cholesterol numbers. Discuss the risk factors that you can change and the ones that cannot be changed.

Quote the Serenity Prayer: *"God grant me the serenity to accept the things I cannot change, the courage to change the things I can, and the wisdom to know the difference."* Discuss answers to the OUTREACH activity.

Ask a volunteer to read the information given by the American Cancer Society on page 77. Ask, Were you surprised to learn that breast cancer is not the number one cancer killer for women? Discuss the lifestyles that contribute to cancer: tobacco, alcohol, poor nutrition,

inactivity, obesity, and sexually transmitted germs. Ask, Is God allowing society to destroy itself? Read Exodus 15:26.

Ask someone to read Professor Phitt's comments on page 79. Compare characteristics of people with type 1 diabetes and those with type 2 diabetes. Encourage members to make changes today that will affect tomorrow and the next generation. To close the session, stand and praise God by quoting together the Verse to Know (repeat several times).

Assignments for this Week:
- Complete Week 10 in Member Workbook.
- Record food and activity in the *Accountability Journal*.

After the Session
- Pray for the members of your class.

SESSION 10

Session Goal
To make members aware of various methods of alternative and complimentary medicines and therapies; emphasizing that Total Wellness is the best choice.

Before the Session
- Read the session options for session 11 (p. 111). Begin to plan for the final class. Involve class members in the plans if possible. Contact these members this week.
- Review previous chapters and Session Goals in order to review the entire book during this session.

During the Session
Greet members and share prayer requests; as requests are mentioned, assign a volunteer to voice the prayer.

Read the Verses to Know from several different translations and remind the group that the price was very costly to God—His Son Jesus. Our bodies are God's temples and we should be the caretakers.

Review the terms listed on pages 81-82. Share the OUTREACH activity; if no one has been involved in a medical study, discuss briefly the ads that appear on radio and television asking for volunteers to join a study. Ask members to share experiences they have had with the CAMs presented in the chapter. Read the warnings listed as Red Flags on page 88. Allow time for questions.

Ask members to review their goals from week 1, and say, After receiving the information in this book, do you need to make adjustments to your goals? Encourage members to review their *Accountability Journal* to see what lifestyle changes they have made during the study.

Review each chapter and discuss the advantages that weight management and strength building have on "God's temple."

Remind members that history can't be changed, but changing the present can improve the future, at least with health matters. Encourage everyone to know the causes of stress and to commit to a quiet time with the Heavenly Father for needed rest.

Discuss briefly how we can fulfill Mark 12:30-31 with the information received in this study: "Love the Lord …with all my strength." Join hands and close with prayer.

Share plans for the final session and encourage members to be prepared according to the option you've chosen.

Assignments for this Week:
• Record food and activity in *Accountability Journal*.

After the Session
• Consider writing a note thanking each of the participants. Mention a specific contribution she or he has made to you and to the group.

SESSION 11

Session Goal
To wrap up this study through sharing testimonies and fellowship time.

Option 1
Plan to meet as a group for a healthy potluck meal. Encourage members to bring a nutritious dish from the *Fit 4 Wise Choices* cookbook if possible. Otherwise, ask members bring the recipes of their dishes to share with the class.

Informally invite members to share what they learned from this study of physical wellness.

Ask members to review the goals they set at the beginning of the session. Have them evaluate their progress toward accomplishing these goals. Remind them that they only fail when they choose to quit. Slow progress toward a goal is still progress. Remember: progress, not perfection, is the key on the wellness journey.

Encourage members to take other *Fit 4* courses to further develop their wellness plan. Close the time together by holding hands and having each person that is willing pray a sentence prayer of gratitude to God.

Option 2
Invite a panel of at least three health and medical professionals to your session (doctors, nurses, dietitians, fitness trainers or instructors, alternative medical professionals, representatives from local health organizations such as the American Heart Association, or representatives from the local health department). Have each professional give a brief summary of their expertise. Then allow the class to ask questions of these professionals based on the various topics covered in the study. Allow the time to be a dialogue and not a formal presentation.

If you choose this option, contact the class prior to the session to prepare written questions for the guest professionals based on their review of the study.

Conclude the session by saying Mark 12:30-31 aloud. Pray a prayer of thanksgiving for each person and their wellness journey.

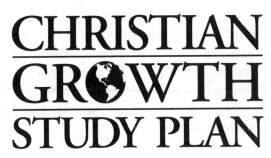

Preparing Christians to Serve

In the **Christian Growth Study Plan (formerly Church Study Course),** this book *With All My Strength* is a resource for course credit in the subject area Personal Life of the Christian Growth category of diploma plans. To receive credit, read the book, complete the learning activities, show your work to your pastor, a staff member or church leader, then complete the following information. This page may be duplicated. Send the completed page to:

**Christian Growth Study Plan
One LifeWay Plaza; Nashville, TN 37234-0117
FAX: (615)251-5067**

For information about the Christian Growth Study Plan, refer to the Christian Growth Study Plan Catalog. It is located online at www.lifeway.com. If you do not have access to the Internet, contact the Christian Growth Study Plan office (1.800.968.5519) for the specific study plan you need for your ministry.

With All My Strength
COURSE NUMBER: CG-0538

PARTICIPANT INFORMATION

Social Security Number (USA ONLY-optional) Personal CGSP Number* Date of Birth (MONTH, DAY, YEAR)

Name (First, Middle, Last) Home Phone

Address (Street, Route, or P.O. Box) City, State, or Province Zip/Postal Code

CHURCH INFORMATION

Church Name

Address (Street, Route, or P.O. Box) City, State, or Province Zip/Postal Code

CHANGE REQUEST ONLY

☐ Former Name

☐ Former Address City, State, or Province Zip/Postal Code

☐ Former Church City, State, or Province Zip/Postal Code

Signature of Pastor, Conference Leader, or Other Church Leader Date

*New participants are requested but not required to give SS# and date of birth. Existing participants, please give CGSP# when using SS# for the first time. Thereafter, only one ID# is required. **Mail to:** Christian Growth Study Plan, One LifeWay Plaza, Nashville, TN 37234-0117. Fax: (615)251-5067.

Rev. 5-02